Praise for Dr. Mark Hyman's THE ULTRASIMPLE DIET

"This simple, elegant, scientifically grounded book confirms the approach to treatment and prevention I have successfully used for 35 years. It is the single best, and the most user-friendly, guide to good eating and good health that I know of. Buy it. Read it. Use it. And enjoy the benefits."

—James S. Gordon, M.D., author of *Manifesto for a New Medicine: Your Guide to Healing Partnerships and the Wise Use of Alternative Therapies,* and founder and director of the Center for Mind-Body Medicine

"Dr. Mark Hyman brilliantly makes the case for "fattening" toxins as an unsuspected source of weight gain and inflammation. His ULTRASIMPLE DIET and lifestyle suggestions will not only cleanse your system, but will ensure continuing weight loss and optimum health for many, many years to come. Highly recommended."

—Ann Louise Gittleman, Ph.D., C.N.S., *New York Times* bestselling author of *The Fat Flush Plan* and *The Fast Track Detox Diet*

"At last a practical, effective approach to diet that is based on sound science rather than hype. Clearly, Dr. Hyman's new program will be truly enlightening to the public and help thousands fight the underlying causes of disease and obesity. Founded on two fundamental principles of biology, Dr. Hyman shows you step-by-step how to eliminate harmful toxins, regain your youthful health and discover the principles for permanent weight loss. If you are ready to start fresh with a clean slate, this is your program."

—Dr. Kenneth R. Pelletier, author of *The Best Alternative Medicine,* and Clinical Professor of Medicine, University of California (UCSF) and University of Arizona Schools of Medicine

"Dr. Hyman's 7-day program is equal parts power and simplicity. If you give him seven days, he'll shows you how to lose weight automatically, reduce chronic symptoms by half, and establish healthy eating habits for life. Finally, a diet that establishes beneficial eating habits for life AND makes you more gorgeous."

—Susan Piver, author of *The Hard Questions*
and *How Not to Be Afraid of Your Own Life*

"In The UltraSimple Diet, Dr. Hyman makes a radical claim, that inflammation and toxicity caused by the standard American diet leads to weight gain, fluid accumulation and a host of physical and mental ailments. Though the science in this area is evolving, the essence of Dr. Hyman's prescription really isn't radical at all: a natural foods diet. Stories throughout the book suggest that this approach has transformed the lives of many."

—David S. Ludwig, M.D., Ph.D., director of the
Optimal Weight for Life program, Children's Hospital Boston,
and author of *Ending the Food Fight* (Houghton Mifflin, 2007)

"Dr. Hyman has done it again—made difficult health concepts understandable and easy to implement. Fundamental to good health is a whole foods diet and toxin elimination. This book makes it simple and the many patient stories of personal success are inspiring."

—Joseph E. Pizzorno, Jr., ND, Editor in Chief of *Integrative
Medicine, A Clinician's Journal* and co-author of the
Encyclopedia of Natural Medicine

Praise for Dr. Mark Hyman's ULTRAMETABOLISM

"Dr. Hyman, an expert's expert on healing, shares his secrets to harvesting your body's potential for weight loss. Reading this compelling book is the next best thing to entering a cutting-edge health program."

—Mehmet C. Oz, M.D., co-author of *the New York Times*
#1 bestseller *You: The Owner's Manual*

"*UltraMetabolism* is a gem. Scientific, practical, and user-friendly, it gives you everything you need to know for creating a lean, healthy body."

—Christiane Northrup, M.D., author of *The Wisdom of Menopause*

Many people saw they benefited from trying this program, but some found the results dramatic. Here are what a few had to say.*

*"I knew my clothes were loose
but had no idea I dropped 20 pounds."*

By day 3 I was more alert and focused than I've been in years. I was never hungry, and after the initial weigh-in, I didn't weigh myself until after day 7. I knew my clothes were loose but had no idea I dropped 20 pounds. I had lots of energy, more drive, and more focus than I ever thought was possible. I slept better than I could have imagined.

**Denise Owings
Donald, OR**

". . . I learned which foods actually help me lose weight . . ."

Often, I would lose weight with the latest fad diet but inevitably gain it back with interest. Because the UltraSimple program only required a week, I gave it a try. Ultimately, I lost 4 pounds in the 7 days (3 more since then) and feel so much better. With this program I learned which foods actually help me lose weight. I'm not as tired as I was every day or hungry (your UltraShakes are very filling). I am confident I will continue to lose and keep it off. Thanks.

**Patty Saburn
Far Hills, NJ**

* All before and after medical conditions are self-reported, and have not been verified.

". . . positively affected my mind, body, and spirit."

At 49 years old I have endured a lot of stress with work, being premenopausal, and being a mom of two active boys who play ice hockey 5–7 days a week 30 miles from home. I have felt depressed and not in control for some time. The UltraSimple Diet positively affected my mind, body, and spirit. After 3 days I felt like I had my old self back. My weight was decreasing daily; I had amazing energy without the use of coffee and just a sense of well-being that I thought was gone forever. Thanks, Dr. Hyman.

Debra Licolli
San Carlos, CA

"I cannot believe it. 16 pounds and 3 inches in one week!"

I cannot believe it. 16 pounds and 3 inches in one week! Obviously, there was a lot of toxic fluid. I would have never known this without your book. I know these results were due to following the expanded program. The supplements made all the difference, and were well worth the money. I was never hungry, and did not crave any food. This week gave me the motivation to want to continue and you gave me the tools.

Diane Rupinski
Woodstock, CT

". . . this diet was very easy for me to stick to."

I am very impatient, and get tired of any type of strict regimen. However, this diet was very easy for me to stick to. It kept me full, and I never had any real cravings for those foods I shouldn't eat. I lost 3 pounds in that first week and was thrilled.

Tina Holton
Orlando, FL

THE
ULTRASIMPLE
DIET

KICK-START YOUR METABOLISM AND
SAFELY LOSE UP TO 10 POUNDS IN 7 DAYS

Mark Hyman, M.D.

Pocket Books

New York   London   Toronto   Sydney

This publication contains the opinions and ideas of the author. It is intended to provide helpful and informative material on the subjects addressed in the publication. It is sold with the understanding that the author and publisher are not engaged in rendering medical, health, psychological, or any other kind of personal professional services in the book. If the reader requires personal medical, health, or other assistance or advice, a competent professional should be consulted.

The author and publisher specifically disclaim all responsibility for any liability, loss, or risk, personal or otherwise, that is incurred as a consequence, directly or indirectly, of the use and application of any of the contents of this book.

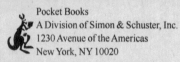

Pocket Books
A Division of Simon & Schuster, Inc.
1230 Avenue of the Americas
New York, NY 10020

Copyright © 2007 by Mark Hyman, M.D.

All rights reserved, including the right to reproduce this book or portions thereof in any form whatsoever. For information address Pocket Books Subsidiary Rights Department, 1230 Avenue of the Americas, New York, NY 10020

First Pocket Books paperback edition April 2007

POCKET and colophon are registered trademarks of Simon & Schuster, Inc.

For information about special discounts for bulk purchases, please contact Simon & Schuster Special Sales at 1-800-456-6798 or business@simonandschuster.com.

Designed by Suet Chong

Manufactured in the United States of America

30 29 28 27 26 25 24 23 22 21

ISBN-13: 978-1-4165-4776-1
ISBN-10:   1-4165-4776-2

*For the millions of people who suffer
needlessly from chronic disease*

CONTENTS

THE
UltraSimple
DIET

CHAPTER 1

Why the UltraSimple Diet?

"I lost 3 pounds right away, my sugar levels stabilized, and my energy level shot up."

My entire life, even after having children, I have been plagued with depression, chronic fatigue, allergies, debilitating headaches, constant mood swings, and anxiety. After hearing for years from doctors that it was all "in my head," I decided to jump on Dr. Hyman's program, because I had nothing more to lose. Immediately after following his instructions, I started to feel calm and began sleeping throughout the night. I naturally started eating less, because I was full and satisfied. I lost 3 pounds right away, my sugar levels stabilized, and my energy level shot up. For the first time, I can live in the moment. I feel better, my heart palpitations are gone, the ringing in my ears has diminished, my headaches have stopped, and my focus and concentration have improved dramatically. This simply happened as a result of removing the toxins from my diet and eating nourishing whole foods. This experience on The UltraSimple Diet has completely changed my life.

Carla Goodrich
Columbus, NE

Could this be you? This was one user of the program, although not all results were this striking. More dramatic results are at the beginning of each chapter.

For more success stories, go to www.ultrasimplediet.com/success.

In this chapter you will learn:

- ✧ The 6 steps of The UltraSimple Diet
- ✧ The 4 additional steps of The Enhanced UltraSimple Diet
- ✧ Why the program works
- ✧ Who I am

We have all the scientific information we need to address the obesity epidemic facing our society and threatening our children and our longevity.

The problem is most of you are not hearing about it. It takes an average of 20 years for new medical discoveries to be applied in practice.

But, you don't have to wait—it's available right now, here in this program.

I have to admit something to you: The term *diet* in the title of this book is a bit misleading. This is really a 7-day health program wherein one of the natural consequences is healthy weight loss as I'll explain in a second.

After working with thousands of patients for more than 20 years; heading the medical department of one of the world's top health resorts, Canyon Ranch, for 9 years; and being the founder and medical director of The UltraWellness Center, I have discovered what works and what doesn't to give people quick, yet safe results for revitalizing their health and achieving weight loss.

And I have the results to prove it, which you can see for yourself by going to www.ultrasimplediet.com/success where you'll find hundreds of success stories from people who have already been through this program.

In fact, throughout this book, I've included comments from

real people who have actually already gone through the program so you can see how well it has worked for them.

Even after looking at these success stories, if you are still skeptical that you can't lose up to 10 pounds in 7 days, you are right—you shouldn't believe it. There are so many false weight-loss claims flying around today that it's tough to believe what works and what doesn't.

The only way to know that it's true is to try the program and prove it to yourself. This program won't work for everybody, but it should work for most, and in many cases you may get the kind of dramatic results I've highlighted in this book.

The real trick is that the same things that make people sick make them fat. In fact, being overweight is actually a symptom of an underlying health problem.

So, it's not really a trick or a gimmick at all—in this program, you'll be working on some of the underlying, fundamental problems that make people fat.

And being fat creates even more sickness and disease—including heart disease, cancer, arthritis, dementia, and diabetes.

The answer to effective, long-term weight loss is addressing the underlying causes of obesity and disease. For most of you out there suffering with weight issues there are two key causes: **toxicity and inflammation.**

In fact, for many of you, toxicity in particular may be what's been frustrating your weight-loss attempts. As I'll explain in chapter 3, you may be carrying around a truckload of toxins in your body that are disrupting your body's natural mechanisms for health. And as you'll see, getting healthy is the key to losing weight.

This can frequently explain why people seem to reach a plateau or "hit the wall" when attempting to lose weight, where, after an initial drop in weight, further weight loss proves to be next to impossible. Just restricting calories is a recipe for disaster and inevitably leads to failure. Unless you get rid of this toxic load, you might find yourself continually hitting this wall.

Take the "Toxicity and Inflammation Quiz" in chapter 2 and you may be surprised to find out how toxic and inflamed you really are. Don't worry; I'll explain what those two terms mean after you have taken the quiz.

The UltraSimple Diet provides a quick-start plan for dramatically, powerfully, and simply addressing toxicity and inflammation.

Dealing with toxicity and inflammation may not only help you lose up to 10 pounds in 7 days, but may also provide you with a feeling of robust health and relief of many chronic symptoms.

Some of you may ask "Isn't it all just water weight?" or "Isn't it unhealthy to lose more than 1–2 pounds per week?"

The truth is that you WANT to lose water weight.

Inflammation and toxicity cause fluid retention. Cleaning up your system for one week, by consuming a detoxifying and anti-inflammatory diet, may help you drop fluid and toxins quickly. This may lead to rapid weight loss, which is both safe and healthy under these circumstances.

Once you have eliminated the initial toxic fluid and inflammation, and you continue to follow my simple guides, your weight loss may continue at a rate of ½–2 pounds per week until you are at your healthy weight.

During this week you may lose both fluid and fat. How much of each varies from person to person.

You may also notice other benefits.

Besides increased energy, you may lose the puffiness in your face and around your eyes, and your skin may even glow. Your senses may be heightened. You may sleep better, have fewer allergies, and more mental clarity. Your joint and muscle aches may disappear and all your digestive problems, such as irritable bowel syndrome and reflux, may vanish.

This will also be the beginning, I hope, of a new way of life for you. Not because I say it is good for you. NO! Your life will change, because you may not only lose weight, have more energy, and feel fantastic, but you may—probably for the first time in your life—have a taste of *vital well-being* and experience for yourself what it means to live an UltraWellness lifestyle.

What Is The UltraSimple Diet?

As I mentioned above, this program is founded on two fundamental principles of biology. To regain health and achieve consistent, permanent weight loss, you need to address the underlying cause of diseases and obesity: **toxicity and inflammation.**

It gives you an opportunity to achieve IMMEDIATE weight loss, but more importantly offers you renewed energy and relief from many chronic diseases in just 7 short days.

But how, you may ask, can you achieve such results in just 7 days?

Simple.

Take away the things that make you toxic and inflamed.

Provide your body with foods and activities that help you detoxify and cool inflammation.

Your body does the rest automatically. It has a natural ability to find balance and heal once you stop doing things that throw it off balance and provide things that put it back in balance.

By eliminating the major sources of toxins in your life—addictive habits such as coffee, sugar, alcohol, processed food, fast food, junk food, trans fats, and high-fructose corn syrup—and reducing toxic stress for only 7 days, your body can renew and rejuvenate itself.

By eliminating the major sources of inflammation in your

diet—food allergens, sugar and flour products, and bad fats—
your body can heal.

Then, by eating whole, detoxifying, anti-inflammatory
foods, the power of the program can take full effect.

Let me be completely honest here.

My motivation is not to help you "lose a quick 10 pounds,"
although that is a nice side effect. My desire is for you to experience in *one week* the power you have to harm or to heal your
body, the power wrong foods have to create sickness, and the
power right foods have to promote weight loss and health.

That way you can make the connection between your behaviors, what you put in your mouth, how you treat your body,
and how you feel and look every day.

I am amazed at how the smartest people don't make the
connections between what they eat, how they live, and how
they feel.

You have the power to transform your life forever by choosing to work with your body, rather than against it.

You see, the primary reason that I designed this program
was based on feedback that I received about my UltraMetabolism program that I outlined in my recent *New York Times* best-
selling book, *UltraMetabolism: The Simple Plan for Automatic
Weight Loss.*

The problem that many people ran into was that they
thought 8 weeks was too long a commitment and never gave
the program a chance. In reality it's not; however, as a consequence of receiving that feedback, I designed this program to
be only 7 days (which anybody can do) to prove just how good
you can actually feel once you have addressed the core problems of toxicity and inflammation.

And as my patients and the hundreds of people who have
helped me evaluate this program have seen, some of the results
can be quite amazing. I had many people comment that they
were surprised at just how good they could feel and never real-

ized that by simply changing their diet, they could feel more energized, sleep better, have better-looking skin, lose weight, improve their mood, and more in only 7 days.

This program will give you the power to make this transformation.

Here's how you do it:

Get Rid of Bad Foods—Eliminate foods that create toxicity and inflammation.

Add Good Foods—Eat foods that are detoxifying and anti-inflammatory.

Detoxify—Drink a special, cleansing and detoxifying Ultra-Broth, and keep your bowels clear during the program by taking an herbal laxative as needed.

Reduce Inflammation—Make delicious, anti-inflammatory UltraShakes.

Relax—Take a fabulously relaxing and detoxifying UltraBath every night before bed.

Reflect—Reflect and write in your journal about what you're learning and how you're feeling during the program.

That's it.

Do it for 7 days and watch the transformation take place.

In fact, if many of you are thinking of this as a "diet" in the traditional sense, you are also probably worried about several things. Remember, this isn't so much a diet as it is a medically designed eating program, and, as such, you won't have to worry about:

Going Hungry—This is not a starvation diet. You shouldn't be hungry over the course of the diet, and you won't be as long as you follow my recommendations. In fact, one of the most common points of feedback I've received from people who have been on this program has been how they actually had too much food prepared and didn't need it all since they simply weren't hungry.

Having Cravings—You're worried about cravings? Forget it! My patients have overwhelmingly reported that their cravings **decrease** when they do the program.

Eating Gross Foods—You also don't have to worry about disgusting or tasteless food. The food options I offer are delicious, and even if you don't like things exactly as I have outlined them in the book, I give you enough flexibility to adjust them to your tastes. Moreover, I've provided a special set of bonus recipes (which I will keep updated) that you can download by going to www.ultrasimplediet.com/guide.

Exercising Too Much—Think you are going to have to go to the gym and sweat for 2 hours every day? Don't worry. Although I always do recommend getting exercise on a daily basis, for just these 7 days, the eating program is powerful enough so that you don't have to exercise if you don't want to.

Waiting Too Long—Frequently people complain that it takes too long to see the benefits of any "diet"; however, remember, by using a medically designed eating program, we are working with the natural forces of your body, instead of against them as traditional diets do, and as a consequence, you typically see the benefits very quickly.

So what have you got to lose . . . except a few extra pounds.

Start the 7-day plan on a Sunday so you have the weekend to ease into it and prepare for your work week. You'll want to also reserve your Saturday to make the necessary preparations, go shopping, and get everything organized for the upcoming 7 days.

Want More Proof?

Simply go to www.ultrasimplediet.com/success and read stories from hundreds of individuals who put the program to the test.

Don't take my word for it. Experience it.

For those of you who want to take full advantage of the healing potential of this 7-day program, I encourage you to add a few things that will maximize the long-term benefits.

I call this The Enhanced UltraSimple Diet.

You simply add the following components to supercharge your health:

Nutritional Supplements—These are designed to enhance elimination and cellular detoxification, and reduce inflammation. Basic lifelong supplementation is also encouraged to support your body's normal functions, and provide the essential nutrients our modern depleted diet cannot.

Liver Detoxification—A special, simple olive oil and lemon juice cocktail to promote liver detoxification by increasing bile flow.

Easy Exercise—30 minutes of walking a day . . . that's it.

Reduce Stress—Simple relaxation and stress-reduction techniques.

Following either of these simple, scientifically proven programs may help you lose up to 10 pounds in one week. But more importantly, it will give you all the tools you need to become the thin, fit, healthy, energetic person you want to be.

A Not-So-Uncommon Story
of The UltraSimple Diet

One day a man showed up in my office who looked familiar. I had seen him at one of my lectures. On his own he decided to start The UltraSimple Diet.

He just changed his diet, and miracles happened. He lost 10 pounds the first week and 20 pounds in 3 weeks.

He is a 32-year-old father of two who works in insurance. When he got married, he was a fit 185 pounds. Over the last 11 years he gained 55 pounds and was up to 240 pounds when he came in.

He worked hard, didn't exercise, ate lunch at his desk, and felt horrible all the time. He was tired of not living life to the fullest.

After hearing my talk, he started the program you will find in this book. Before he started he had a laundry list of symptoms that would have been bad for an 80-year-old, but was scary for a 32-year-old. He was headed toward heart disease, diabetes, and stroke within a few years.

He was exhausted, and addicted to sugar, carbs, and caffeine. He had no stamina, suffered from headaches, sweated constantly, and had lost his sex drive. He had acne, bumps all over his back, waist and chest, bloating, bad gas, reflux, post-nasal drip and congestion, muscle cramps, anal itching, and dry skin. He also had sleep apnea, high cholesterol, high blood pressure, and shortness of breath. Whew!

His blood tests showed a high level of inflammation with a high C-reactive protein test. And his liver was toxic and fatty.

He was a physical wreck and felt horrible. His idea of the perfect meal was a cheeseburger, fries, and coke. Within days he changed his life dramatically by cleaning up his diet, giving up sugar, caffeine, and junk food, and simply eating whole foods. In short, by feeding his body the way it was designed.

He simply changed the type of food he was eating—choosing anti-inflammatory and detoxifying foods instead of the junk food he was accustomed to consuming.

He got off dairy, gluten, eggs, sugar, and yeast—the most common food intolerances or allergens. He didn't even exercise or add supplements.

What happened was remarkable.

Not only did he lose 10 pounds in 7 days (and 10 more pounds over the next two weeks), but his cravings disappeared, and he stopped waking up every morning with a sneezing, runny nose.

His energy and his sex drive increased, his muscle cramps went away, and his skin cleared up. His irritable bowel syndrome and gas went away, and his reflux stopped.

All this in only 7 days.

When the program ended he kept the good habits he created, and was able to continue living a healthy lifestyle.

When he came in to see me, I encouraged him to start exercising, and gave him a good multivitamin, fish oil, and herbs and nutrients to help his liver such as milk thistle, lipoic acid, and n-acetylcysteine.

After 4 months he lost more than 40 pounds, his liver healed, his inflammation went away, his testosterone levels improved, and he was a different person.

Not only did he lose weight, but he got his health and his life back.

Now he won't end up with heart disease, diabetes, and morbid obesity like the rest of his family.

The power of this program is not just a quick-fix, rapid-weight-loss program, but a process for beginning a way of living that can heal a host of chronic health problems, help you sustain and maintain weight loss, and give you your life back.

Just try it! You won't need me to convince you.

Why the Program Works

The plan works for one very simple reason.

For one week you take out all the toxic and inflammatory foods and substances (especially sugar and the common food allergens) from your diet, and replace them with detoxifying and anti-inflammatory foods and behaviors.

Then your body's natural intelligence does the rest.

It is that simple.

The body knows what to do if you simply get out of the way. If you give it a rest and a chance to repair and heal, it will.

You may even discover how bad you were feeling and how great you can really feel, if you address toxicity and inflammation (especially by eliminating common food allergens).

Most of us have no idea how our choice of foods and our behaviors influence how we feel. After all, if we knew what made us get fat or feel bad, wouldn't we stop?

This program gives you a chance to discover just how good you can feel in one short week.

A Little Bit about Me . . .

I tell you these things, not because I have read them in a book, or learned about them through medical research (although there are thousands of studies that support the foundational principles of the program you are about to learn).

No, I tell you these things, because I have seen them work over and over again. They have given thousands of my patients back their health and vitality. And they have helped those same patients lose thousands of pounds.

I have applied these principles for more than 20 years in medical practice, in my work as co-medical director at Canyon Ranch (one of the world's top health resort), and as the founder and medical director of The UltraWellness Center.

I have conducted workshops founded on this plan all over the world, guiding people through the experience you are about to embark on, and the results possible within one short week are remarkable.

You can now take advantage of the system I have developed to help you achieve quick weight loss, the opportunity to reset your metabolism, and begin a different way of being in the world—a way free of chronic symptoms and excess weight, and full of energy and robust health.

And the best part is it's simple, it's easy, it's fast, and it works!

To get started, simply take the quiz in the next chapter to discover how much this program can change your life.

Summary

- ✧ The program works by reducing toxicity and inflammation—2 key causes of obesity and disease.
- ✧ Simply eliminate foods that create toxicity and inflammation, and eat detoxifying and anti-inflammatory foods.
- ✧ Balance, relax, and detoxify your system with the help of the UltraShake, the UltraBroth, and the UltraBath.
- ✧ Enhance the side benefits of the program by adding extra-virgin olive oil, lemon juice, supplements, exercise, and relaxation.

What's Next

In the next chapter discover just how toxic and inflamed you are.

CHAPTER 2

How Toxic and Inflamed Are YOU?

"In 5 days I went from constant pain to almost none."

With a total score of 99 on the Toxicity and Inflammation Quiz, I thought following the program for 7 days could only help. I wasn't hungry at all and felt satisfied after every meal. By Wednesday, I noticed that I had very little body pain, which was my main complaint for the past 20 years. In 5 days I went from constant pain to almost none. Amazing! My Toxicity and Inflammation score went from 99 to 57, a drop of 42 points in 7 days. I lost 3 pounds of body weight, and 1.25 inches off my waist and 1 inch off my hips.

Susan Beadle
Mohawk, NY

For more success stories, go to www.ultrasimplediet.com/success.

In this chapter you will learn:

- ✧ How to evaluate your level of toxicity and inflammation
- ✧ How to monitor your progress over time

How do you know if you might benefit from this program? Because I'm a doctor, the only way I know if something is working is to take measurements both before and after I do something.

In addition to quantitative measurements, I am also interested in qualitative measurements such as how my patients feel, how much energy they have, if they slept better, and so on.

Accordingly, I've designed this chapter to be your home base—the place where you can take a baseline measurement of your vital statistics BEFORE you start the program, and the place where you can return to insert your AFTER statistics.

You will quickly be able to see how much your health has improved and hopefully, as a natural consequence, how much weight you've lost.

I've broken this chapter down into 4 simple steps you can take to track what's important. You'll notice that there are three columns for everything: before, after, and improvement.

I've designed it this way, so you can very quickly see how much you've improved in a particular area.

You have three options for recording your information:

Use the Book—I've included everything in this chapter you need to record the necessary information.

Use the Downloadable Guide—You can download all of these forms in *The UltraSimple Companion Guide* at www .ultrasimplediet.com/guide. The forms and tables you will find there are much larger and easier to fill in, and you can also print them out several times if needed.

Use the Special Website—I've also set up a special component on my website where you can track all of this online if you like. To use the online module, simply go to www.ultra simplediet.com/join.

Here are the 4 important, yet simple, steps to take:

Step 1: Take the Health Quiz

Take this "Toxicity and Inflammation Quiz." The higher the score, the more toxic and inflamed you are, and the more the program may help you.

If you suffer from any of the symptoms in this quiz or struggle with weight gain and are resistant to weight loss, this program can help you regain your health and lose weight quickly.

Please note that this questionnaire is not a replacement for regular checkups or medical diagnoses by your health care professional.

Take this quiz before and after you do the program. Make sure you take this quiz and save your results from both before and after the program.

Toxicity and Inflammation Quiz

Name: _____

Date: _____

Just like an auto mechanic who takes inventory of a car's condition before he tunes it up, you should make a general assessment of your overall health, so you know where it needs improvement. As you complete this questionnaire, be completely honest about how you feel physically and mentally.

Please take the quiz before you start the program.

Then take it again once you've finished the program, and see how different you feel. You might be surprised how many of your symptoms disappear in just 7 days.

You can also use the quiz as a tool to measure your progress for the long term. Take it once a month to check in with yourself, and see if it's time for another week on the program. You might even want to make it a habit do the program once every 3 months, and recharge your batteries.

The form below will make it easy to keep track of your scores on the two quizzes you will take on this program.

Take the quiz first one day before you start the program, ideally on Saturday, since I recommend you start the program on a Sunday, and fill in your scores in the "before" column.

Then, when you have finished the program on the following Saturday, take the quiz again and fill in your scores in the "after" column.

Finally, record the difference between your scores in the column on the far right marked "difference."

The first time you take the quiz (before you start the program), rate each of the following symptoms based upon your health profile for the past 30 days.

After you have completed the week-long program rate each of the following symptoms based on how you feel that day.

Rating Scale

0 = Never or almost never have the symptom
1 = Occasionally have it, effect is not severe
2 = Occasionally have it, effect is severe
3 = Frequently have it, effect is not severe
4 = Frequently have it, effect is severe

DIGESTIVE TRACT	Before	After	Difference
Nausea or vomiting			
Diarrhea			
Constipation			
Bloated feeling			
Belching or passing gas			

DIGESTIVE TRACT	Before	After	Difference
Heartburn			
Intestinal/stomach pain			
Subtotal			
EARS	**Before**	**After**	**Difference**
Itchy ears			
Earaches or ear infections			
Drainage from ear			
Ringing in ears or hearing loss			
Subtotal			
EMOTIONS	**Before**	**After**	**Difference**
Mood swings			
Anxiety, fear, or nervousness			
Anger, irritability, or aggressiveness			
Depression			
Subtotal			
ENERGY/ACTIVITY	**Before**	**After**	**Difference**
Fatigue or sluggishness			
Apathy or lethargy			
Hyperactivity			
Restlessness			
Subtotal			
EYES	**Before**	**After**	**Difference**
Watery or itchy eyes			
Swollen, reddened, or sticky eyelids			
Bags or dark circles under eyes			

EYES	Before	After	Difference
Blurred or tunnel vision (does not include near- or far-sightedness)			
Subtotal			
HEAD	**Before**	**After**	**Difference**
Headaches			
Faintness			
Dizziness			
Insomnia			
Subtotal			
HEART	**Before**	**After**	**Difference**
Irregular or skipped heartbeat			
Rapid or pounding heartbeat			
Chest pain			
Subtotal			
JOINTS/MUSCLES	**Before**	**After**	**Difference**
Aches or pain in joints			
Arthritis			
Stiffness or limitation of movement			
Aches or pain in muscles			
Feeling of weakness or tiredness			
Subtotal			
LUNGS	**Before**	**After**	**Difference**
Chest congestion			
Asthma or bronchitis			

LUNGS	Before	After	Difference
Shortness of breath			
Difficulty breathing			
Subtotal			
MIND	**Before**	**After**	**Difference**
Poor memory			
Confusion or poor comprehension			
Poor concentration			
Poor physical coordination			
Difficulty making decisions			
Stuttering or stammering			
Slurred speech			
Learning disabilities			
Subtotal			
MOUTH/THROAT	**Before**	**After**	**Difference**
Chronic coughing			
Gagging or frequent need to clear throat			
Sore throat, hoarseness, or loss of voice			
Swollen or discolored tongue, gum, or lips			
Canker sores			
Subtotal			
NOSE	**Before**	**After**	**Difference**
Stuffy nose			
Sinus problems			
Hay fever			

NOSE	Before	After	Difference
Sneezing attacks			
Excessive mucus formation			
Subtotal			
SKIN	**Before**	**After**	**Difference**
Acne			
Hives, rashes, or dry skin			
Hair loss			
Flushing or hot flushes			
Excessive sweating			
Subtotal			
WEIGHT	**Before**	**After**	**Difference**
Binge eating/drinking			
Craving certain foods			
Excessive weight			
Compulsive eating			
Water retention			
Skip meals often			
Excess alcohol intake			
Night eating			
Subtotal			
OTHER	**Before**	**After**	**Difference**
Frequent illness			
Frequent or urgent urination			
Genital itching or discharge			
Subtotal			
GRAND TOTAL			

Key to the Questionnaire

Add your individual scores, and subtotal each group.

Add your group scores, and give a grand total.

Then check the chart below to assess the level of your health problem and the potential benefits of the program.

YOUR SCORE	HEALTH STATUS	BENEFITS YOU MAY RECEIVE *
10 or less	Optimal health	Increased energy, improved mood, and weight loss
11–50	Mild imbalance	In addition to the above, you may also see improved digestion, better skin, and less nasal congestion.
51–100	Moderate imbalance	You may experience all of the above as well as reduced joint pain, muscle aches, headaches, and more.
Over 100	Severe imbalance	You may experience much of the above, but to deeply address your chronic symptoms you will need the support of a physician trained in Functional Medicine.

* The benefits for each progressive level of health imbalance are additive. That means, the more imbalanced your health currently is, the more benefits you are likely to receive from the program. For example, if you currently have a moderate health imbalance (a score of 51–100), you will likely experience all of the benefits listed for earlier categories (increased energy, improved mood, weight loss, improved digestion, better skin, and less nasal congestion) as well as the benefits listed in your category.

Keep a Record of Your Results Online

Remember, you can also access this health quiz in the downloadable guide at www.ultrasimplediet.com/guide or in the online tracking module at www.ultrasimplediet.com/join.

Step 2: Take Your Vitals

Although the focus of this program is on boosting your health and then letting your body's natural intelligence do the rest, it IS important to track what you can so you can prove to yourself that the program is indeed working.

For that reason, I've designed the following set of vital statistics for you to track both before and after the program. Once you are through the program, you should see considerable improvements across the board; if you don't, you may want to reassess how closely you followed the program, and if you did and still nothing happened, seek additional medical help from your doctor as you may have other chronic health problems that need to be addressed.

Measurements	Before	After	Difference
Weight (in pounds)			
* Waist (in inches)			
** Hip (in inches)			
***BMI (see below)			

* Take your waist measurement by wrapping a tape measure across your back and around your belly button.
** Measure your hips at their widest point. This should be right below the bones of your pelvis and around your butt.
*** To calculate your BMI, which stands for Body Mass Index, simply do the following:

BMI = [Weight in pounds / (Height in inches) x (Height in inches)] x 703

For example, if I am 5'8" (68 inches) and 165 pounds, my BMI would be calculated as follows:

BMI = [165/(68 x 68)] x 703 = 25

BMI is another useful measurement to give you an idea of your overall weight. Too see a full BMI chart so you can look up your score, simply download *The UltraSimple Companion Guide* at www.ultrasimplediet.com/guide.

Remember, you can also access this table for tracking your vitals in the downloadable guide at www.ultrasimplediet.com/guide or in the online tracking module at www.ultrasimplediet.com/join.

Step 3: Take a Picture!

This step is completely optional, but I've found that sometimes it's easiest for people to see the changes by looking at before and after pictures of themselves.

You'll probably get comments from friends, family, co-workers, and others whom you are routinely around, but nothing beats seeing with your own eyes a comparison of before and after photos.

My primary concern is your health, because I believe everything will take care of itself once you've addressed that. But for those of you who are concerned about your appearance, you might want to seriously consider this step to prove to yourself just how effective the program is.

Tip: To get the best results, make sure you take the photos in the exact same situations—for example, take them with the exact same clothes on in the exact place with the same lighting. That way it'll be easier for you to compare.

I've also included a special section of the website where you can share these photos with others and to get emotional support and encouragement, which always make things easier and sometimes even fun! To see other people's success stories and to post your own go to www.ultrasimplediet.com/success.

Step 4: Make a Video!

This will be fun, but again, it's completely optional. This is something to do once the 7-day program is over.

I want you to be able to celebrate your success and share your emotions and enthusiasm with others, and also to remind yourself just how good you felt after the program was over, in case you need any motivation later on.

To do that, all you need is a digital camcorder, a digital camera with the ability to shoot video, or even a friend who has one that you can borrow.

Remember, taking a video can be a powerful way to remind yourself personally how much you have changed, and it can provide motivation to others to do the same.

To help you structure the video so you can get the most benefit from it, here are some simple suggestions:

You'll want to cover these three items during your video (you can easily remember these as the three "B's"):

1. **The Basics**—State your full name, age, city, state, and the current date (month, day, year).
2. **The Background**—State why you chose to go on The UltraSimple Diet and what you had hoped to get out of it. Feel free to explain what health or lifestyle problems you had before going on the program that you hoped would improve as a result of going through it. If you've tried other programs and they haven't worked, you could discuss that as well. Feel free to share anything else important about your background as well.
3. **The Benefit**—Here's your chance to boast about your success. You could talk about how much better you feel, how much weight you lost, how much more energy you have, how much better your sleep is, how

much better your skin looks, how your test results improved. You can also talk about things you can do now that you couldn't do before you went on the program. This is your chance to shine.

Here are a few tips that will make the technical aspect of this process easier:

1. **Good Lighting**—Film the video in a well-lit area. Preferably have 2 to 3 lights on where you are filming.
2. **Good Positioning**—Film your upper body (head and shoulders).
3. **Good Placement**—Place the camera on a tripod, and avoid sudden close-ups. If you do have someone filming it for you, ask them to stay still.

Does all of this sound confusing? Are you new to video? That's no problem; simply visit www.ultrasimplediet.com/video to get more detailed instructions and see examples of how others have done this.

If you are really into video, you could post your clip to YouTube, Google Video, or even www.ultrasimplediet.com/videos where many others have posted their successes.

Moving On

Toxicity and inflammation are the root causes of our modern-day health crisis—the epidemic of obesity (which affects more than two-thirds of the American population) and chronic disease (which affects 125 million or more than 40 percent of Americans).

New medications, surgeries, and advances in technology will not help us address these problems.

Only by recognizing what makes us toxic and inflamed and

addressing that directly will we find our way back to health and well-being.

In the next two chapters we will explore what toxicity and inflammation are, how you become toxic and inflamed, and how you can reverse their devastating effects.

Summary

◇ The number, severity, and frequency of apparently separate chronic symptoms can give you insight into your degree of toxicity and inflammation. It can also reveal just how out of balance you are.

◇ It's important for you to measure your progress so you can prove to both yourself and your doctor how the program is working for you, and make adjustments if necessary.

What's Next

In the next chapter discover which toxins you are exposed to and how they make you sick and fat. If you are eager to jump right into the program and skip the scientific rationale, you can go ahead to chapter 5. Although I don't recommend you do this since it's important for you to understand what's happening inside your body, it's fine if you are short on time. Please be sure to read chapters 3 and 4 later when you do have time.

CHAPTER 3

Eliminating Toxins: The First Key to Automatic Weight Loss and Health

"I like . . . the emphasis on eliminating toxins that have been built up . . ."

What I like most about this program are these factors: 1) It is intelligent: it fits with all of the latest research—in particular the emphasis on eliminating toxins that have been built up over many years. 2) It does not involve calorie counting. 3) It provides a basis for life-long, healthy eating.

Tandy Camilli
Sanford, FL

For more success stories, go to www.ultrasimplediet.com/success.

In this chapter you will learn:

- ✧ How toxins cause weight gain and prevent weight loss
- ✧ How you can successfully eliminate toxins from your body

Obesity and weight problems are not always related to what we eat or how much we exercise. New research points to the role that environmental toxins play in causing weight gain and preventing weight loss. That's why learning to avoid toxins and to detoxify is a critical component to long-term health and weight loss.

Living in a Sea of Toxins: How Toxins Cause Obesity (and Other Illnesses)

Most obesity can be effectively treated using lifestyle interventions based on a whole-foods, low-glycemic-load (food that raises your blood sugar slowly), phytonutrient-rich diet combined with exercise and stress management. But there are people who do not respond predictably to normally successful approaches.

New scientific research links environmental (external) and internal toxins to disruptions of key mechanisms involved in weight control. This may explain why some people continue to struggle to lose weight despite doing all the right things.

They may be toxic.

So what are toxins and how do they interfere with weight loss?

What Makes Us Toxic?

I refer to toxins in the broadest sense—the sum total of our poor diet, chronic stress, and environmental pollutants that overload and poison our bodies and minds.

This includes toxic foods such as sugar, high-fructose corn syrup, trans fats, food additives and preservatives, pesticides, hormones, and antibiotics in our food supply and water supply, as well as mercury, lead, and other heavy metals.

It also includes toxic thoughts, behaviors, and beliefs that keep us chronically stressed. These thoughts produce a flood of hormones, such as cortisol, that promote weight gain around the middle, increase our blood sugar and blood pressure, and even kill brain cells.

Detoxification is a natural and critical part of our biology. It is the process of eliminating toxins from your body and your life.

Where Do Toxins Come From?

Exposure to toxins comes from two main sources: the environment (external toxins) and by-products of our metabolism and imbalances in our digestive system (created when we break down food or internal toxins). Both can overload our body's own detoxification mechanisms.

External Toxins: The Dangers from Without

External toxins include chemical toxins and heavy metals. The heavy metals that cause the most ill health are lead, mercury, cadmium, arsenic, nickel, and aluminum.

Chemical toxins include VOCs (volatile organic compounds), solvents (cleaning materials, formaldehyde, toluene, benzene), medications, alcohol, pesticides, herbicides, and food additives.

Hidden infections (such as dental infections or hepatitis C virus) and mold toxins (sick building syndrome) are other common sources of toxins.

Our modern refined diet can be considered toxic, because it places an extra burden on our detoxification systems through our excessive consumption of sugar, high-fructose corn syrup (these are the two most important causes of abnormal liver function), trans fatty acids, alcohol, caffeine, aspartame, pesticides, genetically modified foods, and the various plastics, pathogens (bugs), hormones, and antibiotics found in our food supply.

Internal Toxins: Danger from Within

Internal toxins include microbial compounds (from bacteria, yeast, or other organisms), and the by-products of normal protein metabolism.

Bacteria and yeast in the gut produce waste products, metabolic by-products, and cellular debris that can interfere with many of the body's functions and lead to increased inflammation and oxidative stress. These products include endotoxins, toxic amines, toxic derivatives of bile, and various carcinogenic substances such as putrescine and cadaverine.

Lastly, by-products of normal protein metabolism, including urea and ammonia, require detoxification.

So this is a lot of garbage to deal with. No wonder our systems become overloaded and we get sick and fat.

I've seen it over and over with my patients, particularly those who get stuck and can't lose weight. They are toxic, and until they detoxify they can't lose weight.

Can Foreign Molecules Cause Obesity?

External toxins are foreign molecules that enter your body and have a serious impact on your health and your weight. It is clear that these molecular invaders lead to many of the diseases of aging and contribute to obesity.

I have identified many harmful toxic invaders above, but even some seemingly helpful chemicals can have seriously adverse effects on your health. Let's look at a surprising example that will reveal just how pervasive and poisonous some chemicals are.

Beware: there may be toxins in your medicine cabinet.

While most drugs are not truly toxins, certain drugs can have toxic effects and cause weight gain. Psychotropic medications, in particular, have been shown to promote weight gain. MAO (monoamine oxidase) inhibitors, lithium, Depakote, Remeron, Clozaril, Zyprexa, and some antidepressants such as Prozac, Zoloft, and Paxil have all been shown to promote weight gain through various mechanisms.

Chemicals can affect your appetite (and hence your weight) in other ways as well. For example, hormones (such as Megace) are used to increase appetite in cancer patients.

Drugs can affect your weight and appetite for better or for worse, but looking for the magic pill that will make you lose weight is a misguided approach. It doesn't take into account the complex systems in your body that make you hungry and cause you to gain weight.

And it doesn't take into account the fact that some of these pills may be toxic and lead to even more problems with your weight and health.

It is clear that medications can affect our weight and may play a role in obesity for some people. However, they should not be the primary form of treatment for people with weight problems.

What's more, it's important to recognize that, if something as apparently benign as medications can influence weight, then certainly other foreign chemicals, including environmental toxins, can also cause weight gain.

Why Should We Worry?

Why should we worry about toxins unless we work with toxic chemicals or spray pesticides for a living? Isn't exposure minimal?

Unfortunately, these risks are substantial, pose significant public health risks, and can no longer be ignored.

We live in a sea of toxins. Every single person and animal on the planet contains residues of toxic chemicals or metals in their tissues. Some 80,000 new chemicals have been introduced since the turn of the 20th century and most have never been tested for safety or for how they interact in the human body.

The Centers for Disease Control (CDC) recently issued a report on human exposure to environmental chemicals. They assessed human blood or urine levels for 116 chemicals (and there were thousands more for which tests were not conducted) as part of the National Health and Nutrition Examination Survey (NHANES).*

While they found high levels of toxins in some people, and low levels in many more, the study, in isolation, may not tell the whole story. Why? Because these chemical toxins move quickly from the blood into storage sites—mostly fat tissue, organs, and bones—so the blood or urine levels **underestimate** the total toxic load.

Both weight gain (because of stored toxins) and the total toxic load can frustrate attempts at weight loss in the following ways:

- ◇ By impairing two key metabolic organs (the liver and the thyroid)
- ◇ Damaging the mitochondria (the site of energy metabolism)
- ◇ Harming brain neurotransmitter and hormone signaling that affects our appetite
- ◇ Increasing inflammation and oxidative stress, both of which promote weight gain

* "Second National Report on Human Exposure to Environmental Chemicals," Centers for Disease Control. http://www.cdc.gov/exposurereport

Fat as a Storage Depot for Fat-Soluble Toxins

The Environmental Protection Agency (EPA) started monitoring human exposure to toxic environmental chemicals in 1972 when they began the National Human Adipose Tissue Survey (NHATS). This study evaluated the levels of various toxins in the fat tissue from cadavers and elective surgeries.

Five of what are known to be the most toxic chemicals were found in 100 percent of all samples (OCDD or octachlorodibenzo-p-dioxin, styrene, 1,4–dichlorobenzene, xylene, and ethylphenol—toxic chemicals from industrial pollution that damage the liver, heart, lungs, and nervous system).

Nine more chemicals were found in 91 to 98 percent of samples: benzene, toluene, ethylbenzene, DDE (a by-product of DDT, the pesticide banned in the US since 1972), three dioxins, and one furan. PCBs (polychlorinated biphenyls) were found in 83 percent of the population.

A Michigan study found DDT in more than 70 percent of 4-year-olds, probably received through breast milk. With the global economy, we may likely be eating food that was picked a day before in Guatemala, Indonesia, or China, where there are not the same restrictions on the use of pesticides as there are in the United States.

Many of these chemicals are stored in fat tissue, making animal products concentrated sources. 100 percent of beef is contaminated with DDT, as are 93 percent of processed cheese, hot dogs, bologna, turkey, and ice cream.

Cancer rates have risen from 20 to 50 percent since 1970, and asthma has increased 75 percent since 1980. This is no accident.

How Do Toxins Interfere with Weight and Metabolism?

Toxins interfere with metabolism, overload our liver and kidney's detoxification systems, disrupt the brain's weight-control systems, promote insulin resistance, alter circadian rhythms, activate the stress response, interfere with thyroid function, increase inflammation, damage mitochondria (our body's calorie- and fat-burning furnaces), and lead to obesity.

Whew! No wonder our metabolism is jammed and not burning the calories and fat we put in our bodies.

Most researchers have largely ignored the effects of environmental chemicals on metabolism. Still, a few researchers have started connecting the dots linking toxins with the obesity epidemic.

While research linking environmental toxins and impaired detoxification to obesity remains in its infancy, these factors can no longer be overlooked. Detoxification is a central component in long-term, effective weight management and creating a healthy metabolism.

The key biological systems involved in obesity (and all diseases) that are affected by toxins are the neuro-endocrine-immune system (the connection between the brain, hormones, and immune systems), mitochondrial-energy production (how we burn calories with oxygen in our cells to make energy), and free radicals that create oxidative stress.

What happens exactly?

Toxins affect your metabolism in several ways.

First, thyroid hormone function is altered by toxins—the liver excretes more of your active hormones so your thyroid and metabolism slow down. And the thyroid receptors (the docking stations for thyroid hormone) are damaged.

Second, toxins interfere with appetite-control mechanisms in the brain.

Third, toxins promote inflammation, which increases insulin resistance. This promotes fat storage and leptin (the "feeling full hormone") resistance, which in turn prevents your brain from recognizing that you are full.

Fourth, toxins damage the energy production in your mitochondria, the little factories that turn food and oxygen into energy. There are thousands of these inside your cells and when they are damaged, your metabolism grinds to a halt.

And lastly, oxidative stress and free radicals created by toxins activate signals inside your cells to slow metabolism and increase insulin resistance.

For more scientific background and references on this subject, see the scientific paper I wrote, called *Biotransformation, Detoxification, and Weight Loss: Systems Biology, Toxins, Obesity, and Functional Medicine.* I have included this paper in the downloadable *UltraSimple Companion Guide.* Download it at www.ultrasimplediet.com/guide.

Now let's learn a little more about each way that toxins can interfere with metabolism. I want you to understand that this is a very real threat to our health, and one that can be addressed by following the principles of *The UltraSimple Diet* and the guidelines in my other books, *Ultraprevention* and *UltraMetabolism.*

Obesity and Toxicity: Is There a Connection?

Effects on Thyroid and Metabolic Rate

Many people reach a plateau during weight loss. After the loss of a few pounds, it is often difficult to shed more weight. What is it that impedes weight loss and interferes with metabolism?

Research has shown that when pesticides (organochlorines) and PCBs (from industrial pollution) are released from the fat tissue, where they are typically stored during weight loss, they lower your metabolic rate.

These chemical toxins interfere with metabolism in many ways.

To begin with, people with a higher body mass index (BMI) store more toxins because they have more fat. Those toxins interfere with many normal aspects of metabolism.

One serious problem toxins create is a reduction in thyroid hormone levels and an increase in the excretion of thyroid hormones by the liver. This is a double-edged sword that wreaks havoc on your metabolism. Let me explain.

Toxins induce a liver enzyme (hepatic UDPGT), which promotes T4 (the inactive form of the hormone) excretion in bile. This leaves you with less around to do the job of boosting your metabolism. At the same time, T3 (the active thyroid hormone) concentrations and resting metabolic rate (RMR) go down as organochlorine levels go up. You end up with even less thyroid hormone in your body, and your metabolism crashes.

In addition to all this, toxins compete with thyroid hormones by blocking your thyroid receptors and vying for thyroid transport proteins (the proteins that carry thyroid hormones around the body), making it even MORE difficult for your poor thyroid hormones to do their job.

As you can see, it's clear that organochlorine pesticides and PCBs lower thyroid hormone levels, interfere with their function, and slow the metabolic rate.

Toxins Slow Fat Burning, Increase Rusting of Your Metabolic System, and Increase Inflammation

That's not all. Toxins damage your mitochondria by increasing oxidative stress. This reduces their ability to burn fat and calories by inhibiting thermogenesis (or heat production produced by the burning of calories).

Toxins also lead to decreased capacity for burning fat in our muscles.

All this means that your fat-burning factories are not working at full speed.

Oxidative stress and free radicals are both causes and effects of obesity. Oxidative stress causes you to gain weight. The weight you gain causes more oxidative stress. This whole process can be set off by toxins that increase oxidative stress and alter cell control systems that affect the balance of antioxidants and free radicals in your body.

Free radicals send signals that influence which genes in your body are turned on and off—genes that control blood sugar balance, inflammation, and energy production in the mitochondria. All of these actions cause both weight gain and resistance to weight loss.

Toxins may also influence metabolism and obesity by increasing inflammation. They activate neutrophils, or white blood cells, which are a critical part of your inflammatory system. Again, all of these factors promote weight gain and resistance to weight loss.

And there are even more ways that toxins interfere with metabolism.

Toxins Impair Central Appetite Regulation

Besides directly lowering thyroid hormone levels, metabolic rate, and fat burning, toxins can damage the mechanisms that allow our hormones and neurotransmitters to control our appetite and behavior. These signals are finely choreographed and extremely sensitive to environmental influences.

Toxins can interfere with all the delicate appetite control systems that are regulated by hormones and neurotransmitters from the fat cells, the gut, and brain. The mechanisms are complex but well understood scientifically.

Putting it all together creates a convincing picture that shows it's no wonder that we can't seem to control our appetites. We are being poisoned, and our normal system for controlling the balance of hunger and fullness has gone haywire.

Research backs this up. For example, one study examined prenatal and breast milk exposure to PCBs and DDE (a by-product of DDT). Researchers followed 594 children who had prenatal and breast milk exposures to PCBs and DDE measured. At puberty, the children with the highest exposures were larger, and girls were an average of 12 pounds heavier.

In a second study, a group of researchers from Laval University in Quebec found that, during weight loss, people who released the most organochlorines from their fat tissues had the slowest metabolism after weight loss. Their explanation for the decreased thermogenesis (or fat burning)—after taking into account all other possible factors—was the exposure to pesticides.

In yet another study, the rise of toxins during weight loss in men slowed down normal mitochondrial function and reduced their ability to burn calories, retarding further weight loss.

The bottom line? Weight loss seems to prevent further weight loss, and one of the key mechanisms may be the release of internally stored toxins that occurs *during* weight loss.

Hormone Disrupters: Hormonal Chaos

The dance of hormones is critical for balancing your metabolism. Environmental chemicals and heavy metals are well-known hormone disrupters.

Low levels of these toxins—levels far below what are considered acceptable by the Environmental Protection Agency—interfere with our normal hormone balance, including our sex hormones. This may lead to early puberty in girls and an increase in hormonal disorders in both boys and girls.

Toxins can affect many of the major weight-control hormones, including thyroid, estrogen, testosterone, cortisol, insulin, growth hormone, and leptin. They interfere with our stress response (our autonomic nervous system), and alter the normal circadian rhythms that control our eating behavior.

While we still have much to learn about this connection, we can no longer ignore the effect of environmental toxins on weight. It is certainly not the only factor in our obesity epidemic, or in any one person's struggle with weight, but it must be considered for anyone who has experienced trouble losing weight.

Fatty Liver: Cause or Effect in Weight Gain?

Fatty liver is the most common liver disease in America, affecting 20 percent of the population. But the major cause is not medication, a virus, or pollution.

Instead, it is the most abundant toxin in our diet: sugar.

Increases in sugar, high-fructose corn syrup, or refined carbohydrate (like flour, white rice, and potatoes) consumption trigger insulin and insulin resistance. That causes fat to accumulate in the liver cells.

Excess sugar calories also increase oxidative stress and further damage the mitochondria. Damaged mitochondria can't effectively burn fat or calories, which leads to a slower metabolism and more weight gain.

A fatty liver further impairs detoxification.

A fatty liver is also an inflamed liver; it is called non-alcoholic steatohepatitis (NASH), a form of hepatitis caused by insulin resistance.

A fatty liver produces more inflammatory molecules throughout the body, creates free radicals, and leads to more mitochondrial damage.

In short, having a fatty liver makes it hard to lose the rest of your fat.

The solution? You guessed it. Addressing the causes of inflammation and toxicity.

Optimizing Detoxification: A Novel Strategy for the Management of Obesity

So now you know that you are probably toxic.

What can you do about it? You can do a lot!

First, you need to avoid toxins. Second, you must boost your own detoxification systems. That is exactly what this program is designed to do.

High-Quality Protein Boosts Detoxification

Your detoxification system relies on the right balance of protein, fats, fiber, vitamins, minerals, and phytochemicals to be effective. All these play a role in helping rid your body of toxins.

For example, adequate protein is required to supply the amino acids (which are the building blocks of protein) used by the liver to help synthesize glutathione. Glutathione is the body's most critical antioxidant and detoxifying molecule—and one that is easily depleted in the face of chronic exposure to toxins.

Protein also provides the amino acids critical for many of our body's detoxification pathways (methylation, acetylation, glucuronidation, and glycination).

So getting enough protein and the right types of it—such as beans, nuts, seeds, whole grains, and lean organic animal products—can help your body handle the poisons it is exposed to every day and help you lose weight. If you are not allergic to eggs or whey protein, these can be good sources of sulfur-containing amino acids needed for detoxification; however, to be clear, do not use them while on this program.

Be Colorful

Many phytochemicals (colorful plant chemicals) enhance detoxification pathways.

These include dark-colored plant foods such as cruciferous vegetables (broccoli, kale, collards, Brussels sprouts, and cauliflower), green tea, watercress, dandelion greens, cilantro, artichokes, garlic, ginger, rosemary, turmeric, citrus peels, and even cocoa.

The phytochemicals called polyphenols found in berries, green tea, and cocoa turn on genes that help boost glutathione, which is the most critical agent your body has for removing toxins.

So eating a colorful diet full of these detoxifying molecules can protect you, and help you lose weight!

Sweating Out Toxins

Heat therapy is an underutilized treatment in medicine, but one that has big benefits. It helps balance the nervous system, reduces stress, lowers blood sugar, burns calories, and boosts the excretion of pesticides and heavy metals through the skin. Sauna therapy is an established treatment for chemical poisoning.

While more research is needed, a review paper on "thermal therapy" suggests many promising effects, including a reduction of inflammation and oxidative stress, as well as weight loss. In a 2-week study of 25 obese adults, body weight and body fat were reduced after sauna therapy for 15 minutes at

140 degrees Fahrenheit daily for two weeks using a far-infrared sauna. One case report described an obese patient who couldn't exercise because of knee arthritis but still lost 38.5 pounds, decreasing body fat from 46 percent to 35 percent after 10 weeks of sauna therapy.

Sauna therapy has many benefits, including enhancing autonomic nervous system balance through increases in heart rate variability, reduction in cardiac arrhythmias (dangerous irregular heart beat), reduction of oxidative stress, as well as mobilization and excretion of toxins.

Treating hot water with a few simple items you can get in your local grocery store (like Epsom salt and baking soda), and soaking in it is a very powerful and easy way to detoxify your body. This is what I call the UltraBath, and it is a critical part of the program. Later, in chapter 7, I will teach you exactly how to give yourself this luxurious and healthy treat.

What Can You Do to Detoxify?

In the face of today's toxic environment and its effects on our bodies, it's clear that we need more research and practical tools we can use now to help us detoxify.

To protect yourself, I recommend a comprehensive detoxification strategy.*

This should include the identification and removal of infections, increasing blood and lymphatic circulation, boosting the body's own detoxification pathways, improving digestive health and function, and addressing the toxic effects of stress.

This program helps you achieve these goals in a simple and effective way. It gives you the unusual opportunity to allow

---

* Lyon M, Bland J, Jones DS. Clinical approaches to detoxification and biotransformation. Chapter 31 in DS Jones (Ed), Textbook of Functional Medicine, Institute for Functional Medicine: Gig Harbor, WA; 2006.

your body to detoxify and renew for 7 simple days. You will observe remarkable changes in your body and mind. You can then choose how you want to live the rest of your life.

If you want to enhance the detoxification process, I have added a step-by-step program that gives you everything you need to know to completely free your system of these harmful chemicals in the downloadable *UltraSimple Companion Guide*. You can download it by going to www.ultrasimplediet.com/guide.

Summary

- ✧ Toxins can cause weight gain and prevent weight loss.
- ✧ Toxins slow your metabolic rate, lower your thyroid hormones, increase inflammation, slow down fat and calorie burning, and damage your appetite control system.
- ✧ You can successfully eliminate toxins from your body through diet, exercise, supplements, and sweating.

What's Next

In the next chapter you will learn how common foods you thought were healthy may actually make you inflamed and cause you to gain weight.

CHAPTER 4

Cooling Inflammation: The Second Key to Automatic Weight Loss and Health

"I never got bloated at all while on the diet . . ."

I had multiple health problems when I began this diet and also needed to lose weight. I weighed 202 pounds at 5 feet 6 inches tall . . . I have irritable bowel syndrome and was given 2 prescriptions to treat it, but I really wanted to solve this problem without drugs, if possible. While I was on The UltraSimple Diet, I had no problem with IBS at all! I went from daily diarrhea to normal bowel behavior. That was wonderful for me as IBS had really limited my lifestyle. The diet was simple, because directions were easy to follow and foods readily available. It was trustworthy because you were not required to purchase diet products from the author. And it worked! I lost 5 pounds in 7 days! I lost ½ inch from my neck, 1 inch from the bust, ½ inch from the waist, 1½ inches from the belly (Hooray!), and 1½ inches from the hips. I would call that amazing! The loss gave me a real lift in my spirit. And, I needed that! My memory and brain function improved. I never got bloated at all while on the diet. The UltraSimple Diet made it clear to me that it does matter what one puts in one's mouth. What we consume affects us head to toe. I am in control of what happens to my body more than I'd realized. I thank Dr. Hyman for this healthy and simple way to improve well-being and make losing weight simple and successful.

Donna Mielzynski
Morris, IL

For more success stories, go to www.ultrasimplediet.com/success.

––––––––––

In this chapter you will learn:

⬧ How an inflammatory diet, food allergens, stress, lack of exercise, and hidden infections can all prevent weight loss
⬧ The importance of hidden food allergies in health and weight management

––––––––––

You're probably familiar with the pain, swelling, redness, and heat that classically signify inflammation. It's something just about everyone out there has experienced.

Inflammation is part of the body's natural defense system. When your body senses foreign invaders, a specific cascade of events is set off in which your white blood cells and some special chemical messengers of your immune system called **cytokines** mobilize to protect you.

Regular inflammation is a good thing. It helps your body protect and heal itself.

However, when your immune system shifts out of balance, inflammation can run rampant, causing a chronic, smoldering fire inside your body that contributes to disease and weight gain.

The question is, how do we become inflamed, and what can we do about it?

What Makes Us Inflamed?

We live an inflamed life! The sugar we eat, high doses of the wrong oils and fats in our diet, hidden food allergens, lack of exercise, chronic stress, and hidden infections all trigger a raging, unseen inflammation deep in our cells and tissues that leads to every one of the major chronic diseases of aging—heart disease, cancer, diabetes, dementia, and more.

And it's by far the major contributor to obesity. Being inflamed makes you fat and being fat makes you inflamed.

Being fat is being inflamed. Period!

If you don't address inflammation by eliminating hidden food allergens or sensitivities and eating an anti-inflammatory diet, you will likely not succeed at effective and permanent weight loss.

Food Allergies and Inflammation: Keys to Your Weight and Health

A key part of this program is helping you identify and avoid common food sensitivities or allergies. This is a huge part of the chronic health and weight problems so many suffer with. And though they are real and well documented in medical literature, they are generally ignored by conventional medicine.

Part of the power of the program lies in giving your body a break from these common inflammatory foods for 7 days and watching the results: namely improved health and weight loss.

What are food allergies anyway?

When people think of food allergies, they usually get an

image of someone eating a peanut and ending up in the emergency room with a swollen tongue, hives, and inability to breathe.

That's what is called an immediate allergy (also known as an IgE hypersensitivity reaction). This is very serious but not common.

But there is a different type of reaction to foods that is much less dramatic and deadly.

It is called a delayed allergy (or IgG delayed hypersensitivity reaction). This reaction is much more common and creates much more suffering for millions of people. It is mostly ignored by conventional medicine. Nonetheless, it plays a HUGE role in many chronic illnesses and weight problems.

These delayed allergic reactions can cause symptoms anywhere from a few hours to a few days after ingestion. They also cause a wide range of problems like weight gain, fluid retention, fatigue, brain fog, irritable bowel syndrome, mood problems, headaches, sinus and nasal congestion, joint pains, acne, eczema, and more.

If you hear someone say dismissively, "Oh, you just lost water weight," they're right (at first), because eating foods you are allergic to causes inflammation, which leads to swelling and fluid retention.

Getting rid of this fluid by reducing inflammation is a GOOD thing, not a bad thing. It is what will allow your body to start the healing process, so you can achieve permanent weight loss and optimal health.

Consuming a low-allergy diet for one week may help you eliminate the excess swelling and fluid that accumulates in your tissues from food-induced chronic inflammation. Despite criticisms you may have heard about losing ONLY water weight, this is essential for you body to begin to heal and detoxify.

And the side effect is that you may lose significant weight quickly and safely.

Delayed or IgG food allergies are a common source of health problems. But why are they so common? How do we get them? Are they permanent? Can we get rid of them?

Food Allergies—An Unrecognized Epidemic

The old saying goes: One man's medicine is another man's poison. Nowhere is this truer than when it comes to our different and unique responses to food. And nowhere in medicine is there more controversy, superstition, confusion, and religious fervor than there is surrounding the subject of food allergies and illness.

This prevents doctors from helping millions of people suffering from allergic, inflammatory, immune, or toxic reactions to the ordinary food they consume every day.

In my practice, treating food allergies and improving nutrition in general is the single most powerful tool I have to treat, reverse, and even cure hundreds of diseases that conventional medicine fails at miserably. Some examples are arthritis, autoimmune diseases, fatigue, sinus problems, hormonal disorders, obesity, high blood pressure, cholesterol, bowel diseases like irritable bowel, reflux, colitis, and even mood disorders like depression and anxiety.

The psychiatrist R. D. Laing said, "Scientists cannot see the way they see with their way of seeing," meaning that doctors were not trained to believe that food (and particularly food sensitivities and allergies) have much to do with health. Even when research is published that contradicts their notions, they can't recognize it, because it doesn't fit into their world view. I say with affection that doctors are nutritionally illiterate—they were never trained in nutrition.

This is unfortunate because millions of people suffer from diseases and symptoms unnecessarily due to their diet, and, more importantly, because of unrecognized food allergies or intolerances.

We are seeing an epidemic of autoimmune (24 million Americans), allergic (50 million Americans), and asthmatic (30 million Americans) diseases in this country. In addition, 20 percent of Americans (or about 60 million people) have irritable bowel syndrome that is often caused by food allergies.

In fact, nearly every modern disease—from autoimmune diseases, to allergic diseases, to digestive problems, to heart disease, cancer, obesity, diabetes, and dementia—is caused by inflammation! These chronic diseases affect 125 million Americans. That means in the average family of three, at least one person has a chronic disease caused by inflammation.

These problems are increasing in the population at a dramatic rate. And they affect *everyone,* either personally or through the suffering of someone close to them.

Has our immune system suddenly faltered? Do we have some genetic flaw that makes us overreact to foods and allergens that we have tolerated as a species for centuries?

The answer is no, and I will explain why a little later.

The typical treatments for inflammatory diseases (antihistamines, steroids, anti-inflammatory drugs) calm down the immune response, but they never address the causes of the allergy or inflammation. Sometimes a doctor will recommend an air filter for pollen allergies or addressing mold in the environment, or he might suggest you eliminate peanuts or shellfish if you have a life-threatening food allergy. But otherwise there is very little advice about how to get to the root causes of inflammation.

Are All Allergies the Same?

A little background will help you grasp why there is so much confusion.

Conventional allergists and immunologists generally recognize only **one** kind of food reaction. This is the acute or type 1 hypersensitivity—the **IgE-mediated response**—which turns on a histamine reaction. It is a sudden, dramatic allergic response to things like peanuts or shellfish that can cause hives, trouble breathing, and even death within minutes. This is why conventionally trained allergists do skin or prick testing (PRT) or blood testing (RAST) to look for IgE antibodies to foods.

Practitioners of functional, integrative, and alternative medicine have long recognized the limitations of this point of view. Now new research confirms what we have long known— that DELAYED reactions to food are controlled by a **different part** of the immune system (**IgG antibodies and immune complexes**).

These delayed reactions can cause symptoms that start a few minutes to 72 hours after eating, making it very difficult to connect the dots and see that what you just ate is connected to how you feel.

To complicate things even more, the symptoms are often vague. Typical symptoms include fatigue, bloating, brain fog, food cravings, sinus congestion or postnasal drip, acne, eczema, psoriasis, irritable bowel, reflux, headaches, joint pains, trouble sleeping, weight gain, autoimmune diseases, asthma, and more.

New research in the prestigious journal *Science** and in the journal *Gut*† confirm this connection being ignored by the rest

---

* MacDonald, TT, Monteleone, G. Immunity, Inflammation, and Allergy in the Gut, Science 25 March 2005 307: 1920–1925
† Atkinson, W, Sheldon TA, Shaath N, Whorwell PJ. Food elimination based on IgG antibodies in irritable bowel syndrome: a randomised controlled trial.Gut. 2004 Oct;53(10):1459–64.

of medicine. Also see my article "Food as Slayer, Food as Healer" published in the journal I edit, *Alternative Therapies in Health and Medicine** for another perspective.

In my practice helping people treat food allergies and food sensitivities is one of the most helpful things I do.

So what have I found after years of testing people for IgG allergies and teaching people how to use elimination diets to help them recover from their chronic symptoms and illnesses?

While everyone is different, there are some foods that irritate the immune system more than others. They are gluten (wheat, barley, rye, oats, spelt, triticale, kamut), dairy (milk, cheese, butter, yogurt), corn, eggs, soy, nuts, nightshades (tomatoes, bell peppers,† potatoes, eggplant), citrus, and yeast (baker's yeast, brewer's yeast, and fermented products like vinegar).

These foods can also cause acute allergic reactions. But they are rare, generally affecting less than 1 percent of the population. When they occur they are serious, permanent, and need to be treated seriously.

But for more than 50 percent of us, there are some foods that just don't agree with us and take away from vibrant, good health.

How Do You Know If You Are Allergic or Sensitive to Foods?

There are two ways to find out if you are reacting to foods. One is a blood test for IgG antibodies to foods. This is useful and can pinpoint trouble areas, but it is not 100 percent accurate.

The second is a simple and well-accepted treatment called elimination / provocation. This means you get rid of the top trouble foods for 3–4 weeks, then reintroduce them one at a time and see what happens.

---

* http://www.drhyman.com/pdf/food_as_healer.pdf
† Chili peppers have anti-inflammatory properties.

Eliminating foods you are allergic to is the basis for the remarkable results people have losing weight, feeling better, and getting rid of chronic symptoms when they follow *The UltraSimple Diet* or the detox phase of *UltraMetabolism: The Simple Plan for Automatic Weight Loss.*

These programs are based on a simple elimination diet: getting rid of gluten, dairy, eggs, and yeast products. Very quickly—in a week or less—people notice dramatic relief from many of the symptoms they thought they had to live with the rest of their lives.

Usually getting off these foods for a total of 12 weeks and then adding them back slowly will allow you to heal your immune system and gut, because these delayed food reactions are often NOT permanent reactions. They are an indication of something out of balance.

Even a week is enough to begin experiencing an improvement in health.

Why Do We Become Sensitive or Allergic to Foods?

So what is out of balance? Well, it is our diet and the way we live.

The old idea that food is simply a vehicle for delivering energy in the form of calories is giving way to a new model of food—food as information. We are now eating a diet that has all the wrong information—sugar, no fiber, the wrong fats, and low levels of vitamins, minerals, and phytonutrients.

Pile that on top of high levels of stress, use of antibiotics and anti-inflammatories, acid-blocking drugs that alter our gut-immune function, and environmental toxins at record levels, and it's no wonder our systems are out of balance.

All these factors damage the surface of our intestinal lining in the small intestine. This lining, if laid out flat, would be the size of a tennis court. And it is only one cell layer thick. This delicate surface is damaged by any of the factors noted above, all of which damage healthy bowel bacteria, creating injury and inflammation in that one-cell layer of gut lining.

When that happens, we have something called a leaky gut (known in medical terms as increased intestinal permeability).

Since many of our digestive enzymes (the little chemicals that break down our food for us in our gut) are located right on that delicate one-cell layer that is now damaged, we cannot digest our food properly.

Suddenly we have partially digested food particles from normally innocuous foods "leaking" into our circulation through the leaky gut.

And since 60 percent of our immune system is located in the gut, right under that one-cell layer, our bodies react by increasing our immune response and creating inflammation. Our immune system, normally used to seeing fully digested foods (like proteins broken down to amino acids, fats broken down to fatty acids, and carbohydrates broken down to simple sugars) suddenly "sees" foreign (partially digested) proteins.

So it does what it is designed to do—attack and defend! That is how we create antibodies and develop IgG allergies to common foods. This is what makes us sick and fat, toxic and inflamed.

When the balance of normal gut flora (the 500 species and 3 pounds of bacteria in our gut) is damaged by poor diet, stress, medications, infections, or toxins, then our ability to tolerate food we normally eat (what we call oral tolerance) is impaired.

Then we develop IgG food intolerances or allergies.

Suddenly we can't keep in balance, and the normal mechanisms in our gut that help us tell friend from foe—that helps us digest food and break it down—get derailed.

Have you ever wondered why when you eat a piece of chicken you don't become a chicken, or when you eat piece of beef you don't become a cow? It's because we normally take all the "identity" out of the food BEFORE we absorb it by breaking down the proteins, fats, and carbohydrates into their most basic parts so we can reuse them to make our own human parts.

But when you have a leaky gut, the identity of the food you eat remains after it is absorbed. Consequently your immune system recognizes that chicken and says, "Hey, what are you doing here?" and calls out the marines (your immune system) to attack.

So to recap: when partially digested foods get exposed to our immune system (60 percent of which lies just under the surface of our intestinal lining) because our gut is LEAKY, then our immune system creates an abnormal response to something pretty normal—eating foods.

That creates weight gain and *many* chronic health problems.

Finding and Fixing the Delayed Food Allergies and Sensitivities

We can do many things to deal with these delayed food allergies, rebalance our systems, and get rid of our chronic symptoms.

This program will help you identify whether food allergies are contributing to your weight and health problems. It will also help you begin to heal your gut and allow you to repair your digestive and immune system, so you can be more resilient and tolerate a wider range of foods.

The plan is designed to get you started on the road to finding and healing this common obstacle to health and weight loss for so many.

As I mentioned above, there are blood tests that help identify IgG food allergies. While they have limitations and need to be interpreted in the context of the rest of your health, these tests can be a useful guide to what's bothering YOU in particular.

You may consider blood tests for IgG allergens and working with a doctor or nutritionist trained in dealing with food allergies. (See www.drhyman.com/md.php for doctor recommendations.) You can learn more about these tests, where to get them, and how to interpret them at www.ultrasimplediet.com/allergytest.

What are the Top Delayed or IgG Food Allergens?

The top 6 food allergens or sensitivities are:

- ✦ Gluten (from wheat, barley, rye, spelt, kamut, triticale, oats, or anything containing those ingredients)
- ✦ Dairy products (milk, butter, yogurt, cheese)
- ✦ Yeast (found in baked goods, bread, beer, wine, cheese, vinegar, and on the surface of many fruits)
- ✦ Eggs
- ✦ Corn
- ✦ Peanuts

A Special Note on Gluten

Problems with gluten are widely underdiagnosed. The most serious form of allergy to gluten, celiac disease, affects 1 in 100 people or 3 million Americans, most of whom are not diagnosed.

Milder forms are even more common, affecting up to one third of the American population.

While there are tests to help you identify this condition, the only way you will know if this is really a problem for you is to eliminate all gluten for a short period of time and see how you feel.

Then eat it again and see what happens. This will teach you better than any test.

See www.celiac.com for more information and help identifying hidden sources of gluten.

This program helps you experience the effect these food allergens may have on you by eliminating them for 7 days. The results can be remarkable.

If you suspect you might be allergic to any of the foods included in this plan (for example, nuts or soy, which can be common allergic foods but have such significant health benefits I have included them in the program), you may also eliminate them. Cutting out all the top allergens from your diet (as well as others that may be affecting you) for a week or two can lead to significant weight loss and improvements in your overall health.

If your symptoms improve, you can be reasonably sure that your system is sensitive to one of these foods.

See chapter 16 to learn how to add these foods back into your diet and identify which of them are causing problems for you.

Summary

- ✧ Inflammation causes weight gain and prevents weight loss.
- ✧ Sugar, stress, lack of exercise, toxins, and food allergies all cause inflammation.
- ✧ Food allergies come in two types—immediate and delayed.
- ✧ Delayed allergies are hardly ever diagnosed but are a huge contributor to obesity and disease.
- ✧ Elimination of the common allergens followed by reintroduction of those foods can help you identify problem foods.
- ✧ Healing your digestive system can reduce the severity and number of your food allergies over the long term.

◈ Delayed IgG allergy testing can be helpful to identify trigger foods.

What's Next

In the next chapter you will learn the full benefits of the program.

CHAPTER 5

The Benefits of The UltraSimple Diet

". . . this program has transformed my life
mentally and physically."

*I have been sick most of my adult life. I have suffered from
headaches, colds, hives, rashes, and many other chronic illnesses that kept me from living my day-to-day life. At the beginning of this program I scored a 90 and finished the program
with a 14—a mild imbalance. The transformation my life took
over the week was incredible. I had enough energy to walk 30
minutes a day. My hives cleared up. My headaches went away
and for once in a long time I felt I could really live again. I cannot explain how much this program has transformed my life
mentally and physically.*

Jenny Andrews
Spring Valley, CA

For more success stories, go to www.ultrasimplediet.com/success.

In this chapter you will learn:

- ✧ The common and potential benefits of the program
- ✧ Common symptoms you may experience in the first
  few days and what to do about them
- ✧ Who shouldn't do this program

Many people begin to experience some or all of the following after this 7-day program:

- ◇ Weight loss of up to 10 pounds
- ◇ Better digestion and elimination
- ◇ Fewer symptoms of chronic illness
- ◇ Improved concentration, mental focus, and clarity
- ◇ Improved mood and increased sense of internal balance
- ◇ Increased energy and sense of well-being
- ◇ Less congestion and fewer allergic symptoms
- ◇ Less fluid retention
- ◇ Less joint pain
- ◇ Increased sense of peace and relaxation
- ◇ Enhanced sleep
- ◇ Improved skin

In addition, here is a partial list of the problems that can result from toxic overload and inflammation, and thus may be improved with the program:

- ◇ Bad breath
- ◇ Bloating, gas, constipation, or diarrhea
- ◇ Canker sores
- ◇ Difficulty concentrating
- ◇ Excess weight or difficulty losing weight
- ◇ Fatigue
- ◇ Fluid retention
- ◇ Food cravings
- ◇ Headaches
- ◇ Heartburn
- ◇ Joint pain
- ◇ Muscle aches
- ◇ Puffy eyes and dark circles under the eyes
- ◇ Postnasal drip

✧ Sinus congestion

✧ Skin rashes

✧ Sleep problems

Chronic problems with the body's ability to cleanse itself of toxins and reduce inflammation can also contribute to more serious conditions.

If you suffer from any of the following, this program may help you fight them:

✧ Arthritis

✧ Asthma and allergies

✧ Autoimmune diseases

✧ Chronic fatigue syndrome

✧ Diabetes

✧ Fibromyalgia

✧ Food allergies

✧ Headaches

✧ Heart disease

✧ Inflammatory bowel disease (Crohn's or ulcerative colitis)

✧ Irritable bowel syndrome

✧ Menopausal symptoms (mood changes, sleep, hot flashes)

✧ Menstrual problems (premenstrual syndrome, heavy bleeding, cramps)

This program involves a simple and easy-to-follow dietary plan that may address 80 percent of the health problems that affect the average person.

The enhanced program goes beyond that and includes supplements, exercise, and relaxation practices.

Just following the dietary recommendations, drinking the UltraShake and the UltraBroth and taking an UltraBath every day for one week can produce profound benefits (more on these later).

But if you choose to do the enhanced program, you may deepen your experience, enhance the elimination of toxins, reduce inflammation even more, and discover the benefits of deep relaxation and exercise, which may lead to an enhanced sense of well-being and benefits beyond the seven days on the program.

If you want to accelerate your benefits, and begin to develop habits that will support you even after the 7 days are over, then you should do the enhanced program.

You will find the program accessible, clear, and nourishing—a true 7-day detox, rejuvenation, and weight-loss plan for your mind and body.

It works through a simple change in your diet.

The enhanced program adds supplements, exercise, and balances the stress response.

Both work to help you regain a sense of vitality and promote safe and effective weight loss. Choose what feels right to you.

Common Symptoms in the First Few Days

The following symptoms are very common at the beginning of the program and should dissipate within the first few days of the program. Don't worry, these symptoms are indicative that your body is eliminating toxins and are a good sign!

- ✧ Bad breath
- ✧ Constipation (This should be addressed aggressively by following the steps below.)
- ✧ Achy, flu-like feeling
- ✧ Fatigue
- ✧ Headaches
- ✧ Hunger
- ✧ Irritability

✧ Itchy skin
✧ Nausea
✧ Offensive body odor
✧ Sleep difficulties (too much or too little)

These symptoms can occur for a number of reasons.

First, eliminating food allergies like gluten and dairy often cause a withdrawal reaction, much like withdrawal from other addictive substances like caffeine, alcohol, nicotine, cocaine, or heroin. We are often most addicted to the foods we are allergic to. This causes an allergy-addiction cycle. Getting off those allergens can cause a brief, flu-like achy syndrome that may last 1–3 days.

Second, toxins in our digestive tract may make us feel ill if we don't eliminate them. That is why it is important to address and prevent constipation for the whole program (as well as the rest of your life), and why below I have provided a step-by-step program for fixing constipation now and forever.

The last major cause of symptoms is caffeine withdrawal. This may cause a predictable headache, fatigue, and an achy feeling the afternoon after you give it up. In chapter 6, I explain in detail how to effectively eliminate caffeine to minimize the withdrawal symptoms.

The best way to get relief from these symptoms is to follow the recommendations below.

How to Avoid Withdrawal Symptoms

Those who consume the most caffeine, alcohol, and sugar, and those who have the most food allergies, will have the most difficulty initially. In any event, symptoms of withdrawal usually disappear after three or four days.

It is best to slowly reduce your intake of caffeine, alcohol, sugar, white flour, and over-the-counter medications (except as directed by your physician) a week or two before you start the program. (I give you step-by-step instructions for managing this in chapter 6.)

Here are some suggestions for what to do if your symptoms become uncomfortable. These are already on the program, so you will be doing these things simply by following the program:

1. Make sure you drink at least six to eight glasses of filtered water daily.*
2. To prevent headaches, make sure your bowels are clean. If you tend toward constipation, follow the steps to address constipation below.
3. If you are tired, allow more time for sleep.

The following are not on the program, but you can do any of them while you are on the program to get further relief from your withdrawal symptoms:

◇ Make sure you exercise daily to help fight off fatigue.
◇ If you are hungry, have some protein in the afternoon such as a handful of nuts or seeds such as almonds, pecans, walnuts, or pumpkin seeds, cooked beans or a piece of steamed or baked fish.
◇ If you're irritable or have trouble sleeping during the program, take a combination of calcium citrate 500 mg and magnesium citrate 250 mg before bed.

---

* The best water to drink is water that has been passed through a filtering process. Common and inexpensive filters are available such as carbon filters like the ones Brita makes. The best filter is a reverse osmosis filter that puts the water through a multi-step process to remove microbes, pesticides, metals, and other toxins. This can be installed under the sink. It's a great (and cheaper over the long run) filtering system. Water in plastic bottles contains phthalates, a toxic petrochemical. Mineral water or still water in glass bottles is also acceptable.

✧ If you have an upset stomach, drink ginger or peppermint tea. Steep a tea bag in boiling water for 10 minutes, and drink up to four cups a day as often as needed.

Constipation and Keeping Your Bowels Clear on The UltraSimple Diet

The problem I hear people complain of most often when they are on the program is constipation. I define being constipated as having fewer than one bowel movement a day. Many people go less than once a day. Some may even go only once a week. Even if this has been your pattern your whole life, it is NOT normal! It needs to be addressed.

For some people problems with constipation are exacerbated when they go on the program because of the sudden change in the way they are eating.

This may result in an increase in your withdrawal symptoms and make you feel ill. You may even experience achy, flu-like symptoms such as headaches, brain fog, and fatigue.

Constipation may also inhibit your attempts at weight loss, because it sabotages your body's ability to detoxify. Toxins in your gut are reabsorbed when your bowel isn't clear.

That is why it is critical that you clear out your bowel before the program begins, and keep it clear each of the seven days you are on the program.

In fact, I recommend clearing out your bowel at the start of the program even if you *aren't* constipated. This is a good thing to do, because it helps ensure your bowels are functioning properly so you can maximize your power to detoxify.

For that reason, I recommend everyone take an herbal laxative the day before the program begins. It's a great way to make sure your bowel is clear and functioning properly.

As long as you are having one or more bowel movements a

day, this is all you will need to do. You will simply take the herbal laxative the day before the program begins (as outlined below), and you can skip the rest of the steps in this section. In fact, I will even be giving you reminders to do this later in the book, so don't worry about remembering it right now.

However, if you *are* constipated, the steps that follow are of critical importance. They are designed to help you clear you bowel and keep it that way while you are on the program.

If you are constipated, I will refer you back to this section later in the book as it becomes necessary for you to take these steps, so read them now and become familiar with them so this whole process is as smooth as possible.

Overcoming constipation is an important part of your journey to long-term health. Even after the program has ended, you can follow these steps anytime you are faced with constipation.

Step 1: Basic Bowel Care

Note that the following tips are already a part of the enhanced program. If you do the enhanced program, you won't need to worry about any of this, because it's already been integrated.

However, if you are doing the basic program and you are constipated, I strongly encourage you to use the supplements recommended below to help you overcome the problem.

- ✧ Eat two tablespoons of ground flaxseeds a day sprinkled on salads, vegetables, or in your UltraShake. They absorb a lot of water, and provide omega 3-fats and plenty of fiber.
- ✧ Take two to four 100–150 mg capsules of magnesium citrate twice a day. Reduce the dose or stop completely if your bowels become too loose. Many of us are magnesium deficient. Common symptoms

of magnesium deficiency include constipation, headaches, muscle cramps, menstrual cramps, insomnia,
palpitations, and anxiety.
✧ Take 1000–2000 mg of buffered ascorbic acid (vitamin C) powder or capsules once or twice a day. This
also helps with detoxification and inflammation.

These products can also be safely used over the long term
to keep your bowels regular and healthy in the months and
years ahead.

Step 2: Take an Herbal Laxative

As I mentioned above, I recommend you take an herbal laxative the day before you start the program whether you struggle
with constipation or not. This is a good thing to do to ensure
your bowels are clear.

You should take the laxative at 10 a.m. the day before the
program begins. That means if you start the program on a Sunday (as I recommend) you would take the laxative on Saturday
as part of your preparation for the program.

I also recommend you take an herbal laxative every day
you are on the program if you are struggling with constipation
and have not had a bowel movement by 10 a.m. As I said earlier, keeping your bowel clean while on this program is a critical part of the detoxification process.

Common herbal laxative preparations include cascara,
senna, and rhubarb. Take 2–3 capsules before bed.

These should NOT be used regularly as they are habit-
forming and may make your colon lazy. However, using them
for the 7 days you are on the program is perfectly safe. Although if you follow Step 1, you will probably not need it. By
the end of the week your bowel should be functioning properly,
so going off the laxatives should not be an issue.

Step 3: Magnesium Citrate Liquid

If you have not had a bowel movement the day after you take the herbal laxative, try taking one bottle of magnesium citrate liquid. You should need it only once if you add Step 4.

After drinking the liquid you should have a bowel movement within 6 hours.

If you don't have a bowel movement within 6 hours, move on to Step 4. But **do this no more than twice during the program.** It should not be used regularly.

Magnesium citrate liquid is available at any drug store. It is often used to help clear out the bowel before colonoscopies or surgery. It can also be used to clear out the bowel before you start the program, or if you become constipated during the program and Steps 1 and 2 are not effective.

Do not use this without first consulting your doctor if you have inflammatory bowel disease, diverticulitis, or have had recent abdominal or bowel surgery or any type of bowel blockage or impaction.

Step 4: Dulcolax or Bisacodyl Suppository or Fleet Enema

Most people can achieve a normal bowel movement with Step 1 alone. Step 2 can be helpful during a detoxification program such as *The UltraSimple Diet,* and Steps 3 and 4 are rarely needed.

If you still have not had a bowel movement 6 hours after taking the magnesium citrate liquid, you should take a Dulcolax or Bisacodyl suppository or Fleet Enema. Both are available in any drug store.

The suppository is inserted into the rectum and usually results in a bowel movement in 2–3 hours. Use the Fleet enema as directed.

Step 5: If You Still Have Not Had a Bowel Movement

If you still have not had a bowel movement after following Steps 1–4, then you need to see your physician for a full evaluation.

By following the guidelines carefully and ensuring that you have daily bowel movements, you not only will enhance your detoxification process but should be able to further minimize withdrawal symptoms.

Often when we stop eating foods we are allergic to, the reactions can intensify for one to three days. This is common, short-lived, and followed by a greatly renewed sense of well-being.

A so-called healing crisis (feeling very fatigued or achy) can also occur if your system is not supported to clear out toxins. The most important thing you can do is make sure your bowel is cleared out at the beginning of the program and throughout this process by having one or more bowel movements a day. Follow the recommendations above to make sure this happens.

Who Should Not Do This Program

If you fit into any of the following categories, please seek medical supervision and consultation before embarking on this program:

- ✦ Those who use medication for chronic health conditions. (Most medications will be no problem, but many people may need less medication during or after the program. In addition, they will need supervision from their doctor during this program.)
- ✦ Pregnant or nursing women
- ✦ Children under the age of 18

✧ Anyone with cancer or a terminal illness
✧ Anyone with mental illness other than mild anxiety or mild depression
✧ Anyone with hyperthyroidism (although people with low thyroid function or hypothyroidism can benefit)
✧ Anyone with kidney failure or borderline kidney function (best identified by your doctor through blood tests)
✧ Anyone who is underweight or malnourished
✧ Anyone who has anemia or a low blood count

Summary

✧ This program may improve your overall sense of well-being as well as help you lose up to 10 pounds in 7 days.
✧ It may also help to cure or relieve many chronic symptoms and diseases.
✧ Common symptoms of withdrawal from a toxic diet and lifestyle such as an achy, flu-like feeling, headaches, and constipation may be avoided or reduced with a few simple practices and supplements.
✧ Addressing constipation before and during the program is crucial to your success if you have problems in this area.
✧ Though most people can safely do the program, there are a few people who should not do it or should do it only under a doctor's supervision.

What's Next

In the next chapter you will learn how to get yourself ready for the program.

CHAPTER 6

Preparing for The UltraSimple Diet

"I lost seven pounds, my heartburn disappeared, and I have complete pain-free mobility in my lower back . . ."

I thought for sure I would be hungry the entire seven days, but to my surprise and enjoyment, I never experienced hunger or hunger-induced fatigue the entire week. In fact, I frequently couldn't consume the allotted portions as I felt full most of the time. It took a day or so, but once I had the preparation routine down, it really was 'ultrasimple'. After the seven days were up, I lost seven pounds, my heartburn disappeared, and I have complete pain-free mobility in my lower back. My wife and I like the UltraBroth so much, we made another batch after the diet was over to drink as a regular beverage!

Steve Pattison
Alexandria, VA

For more success stories, go to www.ultrasimplediet.com/success.

In this chapter you will learn:

- ✧ Which items you need to eliminate 1 week before you start the program
- ✧ Step-by-step, day-by-day instructions on how to prepare for the program

If you want to get the maximum benefit from the program, you will HAVE to spend a few days preparing; gathering the foods, supplies, and resources you need; and eliminating items from your diet that are making you ill and overweight.

For example, if you plan to start day 1 of the program on Sunday (which I strongly recommend), ideally you would start eliminating caffeine, sugar, and white flour the Sunday **before** you begin the program using the steps below, and you would begin preparing food and supplies for your program on Saturday.

If you can start preparing even earlier than that, all the better. But for those of you who work 9–5, you'll probably find it easiest to set aside your Saturday to do all of the shopping and preparation necessary.

You wouldn't take a trip to Europe without getting your plane tickets, finding a hotel, getting the right clothes, and packing your suitcase before you headed out.

The same is true for the journey toward health and weight loss on which you are about to embark.

So take the time to properly prepare for the program. It will make your transition into the program simple and painless.

Items to Eliminate

One week before you start the program, prepare your body for all the goodness to come by shedding habits that interfere with your metabolism. Eliminating items from your diet in a systematic way may keep you from potential withdrawal symptoms, make you feel better, and jump-start the process to weight loss and vital health.

Over the course of the preparation week you should eliminate these items from your diet entirely. Remember, in some cases they are hidden in places you may not expect. Be as vigi-

lant as you can about reading labels and making sure the foods
you eat do not contain the following:

❖ Caffeine
❖ Processed and refined carbohydrates and sugar
❖ High-fructose corn syrup
❖ Hydrogenated (trans) fats
❖ Processed, packaged, junk, or fast foods
❖ Alcohol

Sugar and Refined Carbohydrates

Eating sugar and refined, high-glycemic-load carbohydrates
(like bread, potatoes, and white rice, all of which raise your
blood sugar quickly) fuels the hormones that keep your appetite out of control. Stopping this process for one week will
change your outlook forever.

Are you having a panic attack right now just thinking about
giving up sugar? You are not alone, and you are probably addicted to sugar. But relax. Despite your disbelief, the cravings
will disappear within a few days. That may seem hard to believe, but it does happen. Facing these cravings is the beginning of detoxifying and rebalancing your metabolism. By
doing this you won't be fighting all your urges and cravings for
the rest of your life.

High-Fructose Corn Syrup

You also need to stop consuming high-fructose corn syrup.

These super-sugars quickly enter your bloodstream and
trigger hormonal and chemical changes that make you feel
even hungrier.

Consuming any type of sugar or anything that quickly turns
to sugar in your blood also causes insulin surges that start a

cascade telling your brain to eat more and your fat cells to store more fat.

High-fructose corn syrup is the predominant sweetener in all drinks and processed foods. Keep a keen look out for it on the labels.

Trans or Hydrogenated Fats

You should also eliminate trans or hydrogenated fats. These man-made fats are completely foreign to our biology. They are very toxic and inflammatory.

Trans fats, putting it mildly, are not good for you or your metabolism. They block fat burning, cause diabetes, promote weight gain, create inflammation, raise cholesterol, and are even associated with cancer and dementia.

Eliminating trans fats will, with one quick change, leave your diet free from almost all processed and junk food (although now many companies are replacing trans fat with other poor quality fats and call their food trans fat–free). If you find yourself thinking there will be nothing to eat, you might need to just take the leap and trust that you won't starve to death.

Trans fats are used to keep foods fresh on the shelf for a long time, because they don't break down. So keep an eye on any foods that come in a package or are processed in any way. And keep in mind that even "trans fat free" foods can have up to 0.5 grams per serving, so if you eat 4 servings from a package of cookies or crackers with trans fats you will still be getting 2 grams of trans fats. Not good. Beware! Look for the word "hydrogenated" on the ingredient list.

Caffeine

We use caffeine to keep us awake and to compensate for lack of sleep, but it's a false energy that ultimately creates more stress in our bodies. It's a quick adrenaline rush. Then we crash. And that's when we start looking for something else to perk us up—like some sugar! Try to get off it slowly, the way I recommend, and you will realize that you were more tired on the coffee than off it (but give yourself a few days to catch up on the sleep that you missed having all those triple lattes).

Alcohol

Alcohol is one of the nectars and sweet pleasures of life, but many of us rely on it to relax, and regular use disinhibits us around food. Ever wonder why you are always asked to give your drink order first at a restaurant, and then you get a breadbasket? It's because if you eat some sugar (in the form of white bread) and drink a glass of wine you will likely order more and eat more. Taking a holiday from alcohol, besides getting rid of additional sugar calories, will help you tune in to your true appetite and prevent you from overeating.

Here is a little math that might make you think twice about those 2 glasses of wine at night. If one glass of wine (or any other drink) contains about 100 calories, then 2 glasses a night amounts to an extra 1400 calories a week, or 72,800 calories a year. If you gain 1 pound by consuming an extra 3,500 calories, then 2 glasses of wine a night will add 20.8 pounds a year to your weight!

Just eliminating sugar, refined carbohydrates, trans fats, caffeine, and alcohol can have profound effects on your weight and the way you feel in a very short time, even if you do nothing else!

START ELIMINATING THESE FOODS ONE WEEK BEFORE THE PROGRAM BEGINS!

To help make this transition as simple and painless as possible, follow the steps below. They will help you eliminate caf-

feine, sugar, and white flour from your diet. These are the items
people usually have the most trouble giving up, and getting
these out of your diet **before** the program starts will make it
immeasurably easier.

How to Eliminate Caffeine in 7 Days

If you have been drinking caffeine for a long time, you have to
get off it over a few days. Minimize your pain and the difficulty
of giving up your addiction by following these steps.

Step 1: Start on a Weekend

Begin one week before you start the program. Ideally you will
start on a Sunday, so the Sunday before you start the program
you would start eliminating caffeine. This will allow you to
take naps as needed, since your body will be recovering from
the caffeine and you are liable to be fatigued.

Step 2: Reducing Your Caffeine Intake

For the first 3 days (Sunday, Monday, and Tuesday), cut your
daily intake of coffee, cola, black tea, or other caffeinated beverages caffeine in half. That means if you usually have four
cups of coffee in the morning you would have 2 cups of coffee
in the morning on Sunday, 1 cup on Monday, and ½ cup on
Tuesday. Doing this helps you wean your body off the caffeine,
which should reduce withdrawal symptoms.

Step 3: Drink Green Tea

For the next 4 days (the remainder of the week) you can drink 1
cup of caffeinated green tea steeped for 5 minutes in boiling
water. You may continue drinking green tea for all its wonder-

ful health and weight benefits. (Note that green tea is an important part of the program.)

You can switch to decaffeinated green tea if you want to eliminate caffeine completely. Otherwise it is fine to have one cup of caffeinated, organic green tea every morning. The caffeine is minimal and the health benefits are great.

Step 4: Take Vitamin C

Throughout this process I recommend taking 1000–2000 mg of buffered pure ascorbic acid (vitamin C) powder or capsules. This may help you detoxify and balance your system.

Step 5: Drink Plenty of Clean Water

You should also drink at least 6–8 glasses of filtered water a day. You should do this regardless of whether or not you are getting off caffeine, but it is especially important for this process because it will keep your body well hydrated and can reduce headaches, constipation, and flush toxins out of your system.

How to Eliminate Sugar and White Flour

Eliminating sugar is hard, because it's an addiction. But the physical cravings dissipate quickly once you stop eating it. Here are some tips for how you can successfully do this.

- ✧ Start 5–7 days before you begin the program—you will not regret this! It will make your transition into the program easier. I would recommend starting the same day you cut your caffeine intake in half (the Sunday before you start the program).
- ✧ The tried-and-true method from my experience with

thousands of patients: Go cold turkey from all white flour and sugar products. (Don't cheat—it will only make it worse!)

✧ Include protein for breakfast, such as nuts, seeds, nut butters, or a protein shake. Once you are on the program you will have plenty of protein for breakfast with the UltraShake.

✧ Combine "good" protein, "good" fat, and "good" carbs at each meal. (Good fats are fish, extra-virgin olive oil, olives, nuts, seeds, and avocados. Good carbs are beans, vegetables, whole grains, and fruit. Good proteins are fish, organic eggs, small amounts of lean poultry, nuts, soy, whole grains, and legumes.)

✧ Don't go low fat. Consume olive oil, olives, nuts, seeds, and avocados every day. Despite commonly held beliefs these fats are NOT fattening.

✧ Eat every 3 hours. Snack on nuts and seeds such as almonds, walnuts, or pumpkin seeds (raw or dry roasted only). 1 serving is a handful or 10–12 nuts.

✧ Drink at least 6–8 glasses of filtered water a day.

In addition to eliminating the items above, there are a few other things you should prepare before you start the program. Preparation is the key to your success on the program, so follow the steps and recommendations below as carefully as you can to ensure the results you are looking for.

Items to Prepare

I **strongly** encourage you to get all the supplies you need, prepare some food, and get organized in advance of starting the program. It will make your week easier, more fun, and more effective.

Here's what to do:

Go shopping. Get all the food you need. Get a blender if you need it for the UltraShake. Get the supplies for your UltraBath. Order or get the supplements you will need if you are doing the enhanced program.

Prepare some food in advance. Cook your brown rice. Chop enough vegetables for a few days at a time. Cook up some UltraBroth and have it ready. It will all store in airtight containers for 2–3 days in the fridge.

Start the day before the program (Saturday), and prepare food for the first four days of the program (Sunday, Monday, Tuesday, and Wednesday). Then set aside some time on Wednesday evening to prepare for the last three days of the program (Thursday, Friday, and Saturday).

By getting all the ingredients ahead of time and spending some time prepping the items to be cooked as prescribed above, you will minimize the amount of time you spend in your kitchen during the week and make it much easier to follow the program.

If you work, I have included some tips in chapter 7 for making the program easier to integrate into your schedule. Review these tips. They should make your preparation process a bit easier.

Get ready! You are about to take a journey toward health with no return ticket!

The following checklist will help you start that journey. In it I have broken down all of your preparation day by day. Start one week before you begin the program and check off each item as you achieve your goals.

If you don't want to write in your book, you can download the following checklist at www.ultrasimplediet.com/guide. That way you can print it from your computer and even post in on your fridge to make sure you stay on track during your preparation week.

Preparing for the Program

Sunday
(One Week Before You Start the Program)

- [ ] I have decided to commit to the program for 7 days.
- [ ] I have gone "cold turkey" and cut out sugar and white and wheat flour from my diet.
- [ ] I have cut my normal caffeine intake in half.
- [ ] I have taken 1000–2000 mg of buffered pure ascorbic acid (vitamin C) powder or capsules to support my detoxification process as I eliminate caffeine.
- [ ] I have reviewed my schedule and canceled any unnecessary activities during the program.
- [ ] I have informed family, close friends, and, as appropriate, colleagues that I will be doing this program and may be less available than normal.
- [ ] I have informed family, close friends, and, as appropriate, colleagues that I will be doing this program and would like their support.
- [ ] **Optional:** I have downloaded *The UltraSimple Companion Guide* to make my experience on the program that much easier by going to www.ultrasimplediet.com/guide.

Monday and Tuesday

- [ ] I have reduced my caffeine intake to half of what it was the day before.
- [ ] I have taken 1000–2000 mg of buffered pure ascorbic acid (vitamin C) powder or capsules to support my detoxification process as I eliminate caffeine.
- [ ] I continue to refrain from sugar and white flour.

Wednesday and Thursday

- [ ] I have completely eliminated caffeine and am drinking green tea instead.

- [ ] I have taken 1000–2000 mg of buffered pure ascorbic acid (vitamin C) powder or capsules to support my detoxification process as I eliminate caffeine.
- [ ] I continue to refrain from sugar and white flour.

Friday

- [ ] I am continuing to refrain from caffeine and am drinking green tea in its place.
- [ ] I have taken 1000–2000 mg of buffered pure ascorbic acid (vitamin C) powder or capsules to support my detoxification process as I eliminate caffeine.
- [ ] I continue to refrain from sugar and white flour.

Saturday
(One Day Before the Program)

- [ ] I am continuing to refrain from caffeine and am drinking green tea in its place.
- [ ] I have taken 1000–2000 mg of buffered pure ascorbic acid (vitamin C) powder or capsules to support my detoxification process as I eliminate caffeine.
- [ ] I continue to refrain from sugar and white flour.
- [ ] I have gone through my kitchen and removed (if possible) processed and junk foods, all oils except olive oil, beverages containing sugars or caffeine, dairy products, and anything else not on this program.
- [ ] (If the above is not possible) I have set aside a special area in the kitchen and refrigerator for my foods and supplements and my family/roommates know not to touch them!
- [ ] I have started shopping for the items I need to do the program. (See the shopping list in chapter 7 to identify exactly what you need to buy.)
- [ ] I have purchased the ingredients for my UltraBath.
- [ ] I have purchased enough food for the program.
- [ ] I have purchased supplements (if doing the enhanced program) for the week.

☐ I have made sure that I will have enough filtered water for one week of the program.

☐ I have taken the "before" health quiz in chapter 2.

☐ I have taken all of my measurements (weight, waist, hip, and BMI) and recorded them in the chart in chapter 2.

☐ I have taken my herbal laxative to clear out my bowel.

☐ (If you take the herbal laxative and it doesn't result in a bowel movement in 6 hours) I have followed the steps in chapter 5 for overcoming constipation and properly emptying my bowels.

☐ **Optional:** I took my "before" picture so I can see just how powerful this program is with my own eyes.

☐ I have done the journaling exercise for before the program begins. (See below.)

Sunday

The Program Begins

A Reminder about Constipation

Remember, if you are constipated (that is, if you don't have a regular bowel movement one or more times a day), you will need to follow the instructions for overcoming constipation and properly emptying your bowels in chapter 5 the day before the program begins.

You may also need to continue using those steps each day you are on the program if your problems with constipation persist.

Please refer to the section titled "Constipation and Keeping Your Bowels Clear on The UltraSimple Diet" in chapter 5 for more details and a reminder of what you need to do.

Journaling: Keeping Track of Your Progress and Experience During the Program

Journaling is a powerful technique for connecting to what is important to you and helping you find your inner guidance system. You know more than you think about yourself and your life. You have many of the answers you need within you. Studies have proven that the power of journaling reduces stress and inflammation and has a profound impact on health.

I encourage journaling every day you are on the program. It will help you keep track of your progress, notice the difficulties and benefits you experience, and help you identify more clearly how the choices you make (or don't) affect how you feel.

Though you may want to skip this part of the program, the process of reflecting and writing down what you feel and experience and connecting the dots can be a powerful catalyst to make the changes you experience last a lifetime.

Give yourself that gift.

In chapters 9–15 I have broken down the program into a step-by-step set of instructions you follow each day you are on the program. In those chapters I have included journaling exercises to help you reflect on your experience that day.

For an easy way to keep track of all this (and to have a place to keep your responses) go to www.ultrasimple diet.com/guide and download *The UltraSimple Companion Guide*, where I have included all of the journaling exercises in this book. I've also added a journaling feature to the online community so you can keep track of all of this online. Go to www.ultrasimplediet/join to get access to this feature for free.

I recommend you do this journaling BEFORE you start the program:

❖ List your three most physically toxic behaviors (e.g., smoking, not resting, eating sweets, eating unconsciously, choosing poor-quality foods).

❖ List your three most toxic habits of mind (e.g., procrastinating, moodiness, low self-esteem).

❖ List your three most toxic relationships. What purpose do they serve? What prevents you from giving them up?

❖ What would your life would look and feel like without these behaviors, habits, and relationships?

Now it's time to get started with the program.

_____

Summary

❖ During the week before you start the program, you will eliminate sugar, refined carbohydrates, high-fructose corn syrup, trans fats, caffeine, and alcohol.

❖ You can prevent withdrawal symptoms from eliminating caffeine and sugar by following a few simple steps.

❖ Preparation is the key to success on the program.

❖ Journaling can help you track your progress and help you maintain the healthy changes you made during the program.

What's Next

Next you will find a step-by-step guide to following the program.

CHAPTER 7

The UltraSimple Diet—The Plan

"The ease of the plan and all the compliments from others keep me going on my way to health."

Doing the program, I lost 8 pounds and 2 inches off my waist and 3 inches off my hips. More important than the numbers is how good I feel. I am sleeping better than I imagined I could and I am actually waking up refreshed and ready for my day. My irritability and frustration level has dropped considerably. For the first time in a long time, I finally have the strength to be proactive in my life instead of just reactive. I felt so good doing the program that I have continued eating in the same manner . . . I truly believe that The UltraSimple Diet was just the jump start I needed to get going taking care of myself. The ease of the plan and all the compliments from others keep me going on my way to health.

Kathie Jacoby
Harvard, MA

For more success stories, go to www.ultrasimplediet.com/success.

In this chapter you will learn:

❖ Foods to avoid and foods to enjoy
❖ The step-by-step meal plan
❖ Cooking and preparation suggestions

♦ Making the program work on a busy schedule
♦ Recipes for the UltraShake, the UltraBroth, and the
   UltraBath

The foundation of the plan is actually quite simple.

Avoid the foods and substances that cause toxicity and inflammation.

Enjoy detoxifying and anti-inflammatory foods.

You should not be hungry.

Be sure to eat enough food and shakes to feel gently satisfied but not full.

Your body does the rest.

For those who want additional benefits, I have created the
enhanced version of the program. It includes a plan for supplements, exercise, and stress management.

80 percent of the benefits will likely come from simply
changing how you eat for one week. An additional 20 percent
benefit may come from the enhanced program. If you are a little more unhealthy, have more weight to lose, have a little more
time, or want to invest more up front in your health and well-
being, then do the enhanced version of the program.

That's it—it's that simple.

Here are the basic principles. What foods to avoid, which
ones to enjoy, a shopping list, and a basic plan for each day.

Foods and Substances to Avoid for 7 Days

During the program, you will avoid the following foods. You
will do this effortlessly by simply eating the foods on the program instead. That means you don't have to worry about NOT
eating these foods so long as you simply follow the guidelines
for what TO eat, as those guidelines already avoid these foods.

The program is designed to take all the thinking and choosing out of your life for one week so you can experience its dramatic benefits.

This list is simply to remind you of the toxic and inflammatory foods that most of us consume on a daily basis.

Some of the fruits and vegetables, and even eggs and meat listed here, may NOT be a problem for some of you, but the only way to find out is to stop ALL of them for one week and listen to what your body tells you.

Do you feel better? Do you get sick when you eat them? Pay attention. Your body has much to teach you if you listen.

- ✧ Sugar (white sugar, cane sugar, dehydrated cane juice, brown sugar, honey, maple syrup, high-fructose corn syrup, sucrose, glucose, maltose, dextrose, lactose, corn syrup, and white grape juice concentrate)
- ✧ Sugar alcohols such as sorbitol, mannitol, xylitol, and maltitol
- ✧ Artificial sweeteners like aspartame, etc.
- ✧ Natural sweeteners like Stevia (Although this may be fine in the long run, in the short run it stimulates sweet cravings and will sabotage your efforts.)
- ✧ Alcohol
- ✧ Caffeine (coffee, tea, sodas, except for green tea)
- ✧ Citrus fruits and juices (except lemon juice, unless you are allergic to it)
- ✧ Yeast (baker's and brewer's, fermented foods like vinegar)*
- ✧ Dairy products (milk, butter, yogurt, cheese)*

---

* The most common food allergens are dairy, gluten, eggs, corn, yeast, and peanuts. Soy and nuts can be allergens for some people, but they have so many benefits, that I include them in my program. If you are sensitive to soy or particular nuts, replace them with other beans, nuts, seeds, fish, or lean poultry.

◇ Eggs*
◇ Gluten* (See www.celiac.com for a comprehensive
   list of gluten-containing foods. It is hidden in many
   foods, including anything containing wheat, barley,
   rye, spelt, kamut, triticale, and most oats.)
◇ Corn*
◇ Beef, pork, lamb, or other meat except organic
   poultry
◇ Nightshades (tomatoes, potatoes, eggplant, bell pep-
   pers)
◇ Peanuts*
◇ Refined oils and hydrogenated fats such as marga-
   rine, and almost every processed food in the super-
   market. Even foods labeled "trans fat free" can have
   0.5 gram per serving according to the new govern-
   ment regulations.
◇ Stimulants (these include decongestants, diet pills,
   ephedra, ma huang, and yerba maté)
◇ All flour products
◇ Processed foods or food additives (check labels
   carefully!)
◇ Fast Food
◇ Junk Food
◇ Any foods that come in a box, package, can or are
   commercially prepared that are filled with chemicals, preservatives, and other unnatural ingredients
   to make them shelf-stable.

Foods You Will Enjoy

Here are the foods you will eat on the program:

◇ Filtered water (six to eight glasses per day)
◇ Fish, especially small, nonpredatory species such as

　　　　sardines, herring, wild salmon, black cod or sable
　　　　fish, sole, and cod
✧ Lean white meat chicken breasts (preferably or-
　　ganic)
✧ Fresh or frozen noncitrus fruits, ideally berries only
　　(preferably organic)
✧ Fresh vegetables (preferably organic)
✧ Fresh vegetable broth (three to four cups per day)
✧ Legumes (lentils, navy beans, adzuki beans, mung
　　beans, tofu, and others)
✧ Brown rice
✧ Nuts and seeds (almonds, walnuts, pecans, macada-
　　mia nuts, and pumpkin seeds)
✧ Flaxseeds (ground, preferably organic)
✧ Lemons (preferably organic—don't buy presqueezed
　　lemon juice)

The UltraSimple Diet Made Simple!

Now that you understand how to prepare yourself for the program, you know which foods to avoid and which to enjoy, and
you have learned about all the different foods and vegetables
you can eat, I want to introduce you to the basic meal plan you
will follow every day for 7 days.

I *strongly* encourage you to start the program on a Sunday
to make sure you have everything down before the work week
starts. You want to stack the deck for success!

Follow the plan as best you can. It is important to have the
snacks and broth in between. It will keep you feeling balanced
and satisfied. You can even buy a thermos and have the broth
hot all day!

That doesn't mean you *have* to eat every single thing listed
below. Don't stuff yourself. There is so much food on this program that the only danger you face is making yourself too full!

Don't overdo it. Just eat until you are gently satisfied at each meal.

If you'd like to discover dozens of additional tips that other people who have successfully gone through the program have suggested, you can access those by joining the online community at www.ultrasimplediet.com/join, where you also will be able to track all of your progress, write in your journal, and more.

Here's the program!

The UltraSimple Meal Plan

Please note, cooking and preparation instructions follow below.

Breakfast (7-9 a.m.)

✧ Lemon juice (from ½ lemon) and hot water
✧ 1 cup of decaf or caffeinated green tea steeped in hot water for 5 minutes (You may also have the green tea later in the day. Limit your intake to 2 cups a day.)
✧ UltraShake
✧ If no bowel movement by 10 in the morning, take 2 capsules of tablets of an herbal laxative*

Morning Snack (10-11 a.m.)

✧ 1 cup UltraBroth
✧ Another UltraShake (if you are hungry)

---

* More information about how to take herbal laxatives can be found in chapter 5. You will also find more specific recommendations about the types of herbal laxatives you might consider in *The UltraSimple Companion Guide*. See www.ultrasimple.com/guide for more details.

Lunch (12–1 p.m.)

✧ 2 cups or more of steamed or lightly sautéed veggies
(You should eat enough to feel gently satisfied.)
✧ ½ cup cooked brown rice
✧ ½ cup fruit or berries for dessert (Either here or
at dinner, not both, and only 1–2 times during the
7-day program.)
✧ UltraShake (optional)

Afternoon Snack (2–3 p.m.)

✧ 1 cup UltraBroth
✧ UltraShake (if you are hungry)

Dinner (5–7 p.m.)

✧ 4–6 ounces of fish or chicken breasts cooked with
olive oil and lemon juice OR 4 to 6 ounces of tofu or
legumes* (These can be canned but rinse them *well*.)
I encourage you to spice up your meals with rosemary, cilantro, ginger, garlic, turmeric, or curry, and
sea salt.
✧ 2 cups or more of steamed or lightly sautéed veggies
(You should eat enough to feel gently satisfied.)
✧ ½ cup cooked brown rice
✧ 1 cup UltraBroth

---

* Beans can be prepared quickly and easily by opening a can of white can-
nellini beans and adding it to ½ cup of chopped onions sautéed in 1–2 tbsp.
extra-virgin olive oil and fresh rosemary. Season with a pinch of sea salt
and you have a delicious Tuscan bean dish in minutes.

Alternatives Options for People with
Special Needs or Desires

The meal plan as outlined above is meant to keep the program as simple and straightforward as possible. I developed it this way to keep preparation time down, and make it fit the schedule of a typical working person.

However, over the years I have found that some people like to have alternatives to this plan.

As long as you stick to a few basic principles (like being rigorous about which foods you enjoy and which ones you avoid), this program affords enough flexibility to accommodate anyone's desires.

To give you a sense of how flexible the plan is, and to address the most common questions and suggestions I have heard about the program, I would like to offer a few of the alternatives that exist below.

All of this is outlined in greater detail in *The UltraSimple Companion Guide*. You can download it at www.ultrasimple diet.com/guide for more details.

The Hot Breakfast Option

The UltraShake is easy to prepare, delicious, and full of powerful nutrients that may help you reduce inflammation and detoxify your body.

However, some people prefer to have a hot breakfast in the morning, especially if they are doing the program in the winter in an area that is extremely cold. In these circumstances it can be a little daunting to face drinking a cold shake before going off to work.

The first thing you can try is adding 1 cup of UltraBroth to your breakfast menu. This might do the trick, and will keep you from preparing too many additional items.

If the UltraBroth in the morning does not do the trick, there are at least 3 hot breakfast alternatives you could try.

⟡ Hot rice cereal with almonds, walnuts, pecans, flax-seeds, and/or fruit.
⟡ Tofu scramble with veggies and brown rice
⟡ Leftovers from the night before. I know fish, rice, and broth might sound like a strange breakfast, but it's actually quite delicious!

You can get recipes for all of these delicious alternatives by going to www.ultrasimple.com/guide and downloading *The UltraSimple Companion Guide.*

Trading Lunch and Dinner

Different people have different desires about when they eat their "big meal."

It isn't critical that you eat the items on the menu at a specific time of day.

That means you can eat the lunch menu at dinner or the dinner menu at lunch, whatever is most convenient for you. Remember, if you prepare your food the night before, you can take it with you to work and just heat it up.

More Snack Options

The snack options outlined above are designed to keep the program as simple as possible while offering you the greatest possible health benefits over the course of the week.

However, there are some alternatives you can employ here as well if drinking another cup of UltraBroth or UltraShake seems like too much some days.

Here are a few things you can try:

⬧ Raw veggies and hummus
⬧ Nuts
⬧ Steamed vegetables
⬧ The Tuscan bean dish that I describe on page 91
⬧ Chickpeas with olive oil, lemon, salt, and pepper

You can find more details about how to prepare these snacks as well as others in *The UltraSimple Companion Guide*. See www.ultrasimple.com/guide for more details.

Making the Program Work on a Busy Schedule

I know this may seem like a lot to do when you already have a busy schedule. But it's worth it. The difference you will see and feel is well worth the time investment you make in the program.

Nonetheless, I want to make this program as easy as possible to follow even if you do work full-time (or more) and juggle a thousand other responsibilities. Here's what I recommend.

Adjust the meal plan to your schedule. If you work early or late, you can adjust the meal plan to fit your schedule. Just make sure you have all of the meals and snacks. They should be 2–3 hours apart.

If you eat out, be careful. While I recommend you avoid eating out on the program, I understand that this is sometimes impossible. Some people are obligated to go to business luncheons, for example. In that case, I recommend you follow these guidelines when eating out:

1. Ask for grilled fish or chicken.
2. Ask for a large plate of vegetables steamed, or sautéed in olive oil with a side of sliced lemons and olive oil.
3. You may have a salad, but have them skip the

dressing and ask for extra-virgin olive oil and sliced
lemons.

Consider alternatives. If you find it difficult to make (or eat)
the shake or broth, you can use the alternatives outlined above
as well as those in the recipes that follow, and the recommendations in the downloadable guide at www.ultrasimplediet
.com/guide.

Plan for 2 days of cooking. Cook the day before the program
starts (Saturday) and on day 4 (Wednesday).

Prepare all your broth in advance. On Saturday (the day before the program starts), prepare enough broth for the whole
week. Keep half in the fridge in a glass container. Freeze the
other half in a glass container. Thaw it on Tuesday or Wednesday when you need it.

The broth recipe lasts for 2 days. Simply multiply the quantities by 3–4 to have enough for the whole week.

Heat it up on the stove or in a microwave (though I don't
encourage it) or buy a large thermos and keep it with you
all day.

Though it is less desirable, you can use organic vegetable
broth from Pacific or Imagine Foods.

Make extra brown rice. Make rice twice during the week—on
the day before the program starts and on day 4 of the program.
On Saturday (the day before you start the program), cook
2 cups of raw rice with 4 cups of filtered water, 1 tbsp. of olive
oil and ½ tsp. of sea salt (See cooking suggestions below).
Keep it in the fridge and heat up as needed. Then do the same
thing again on day 4 (Wednesday).

Prepare vegetables in advance. Prepare enough for ½ the
week on Saturday or the day before you start the program. You
can either steam them all and keep in Ziploc bags, or preferably

keep them raw and steam them in the morning (this will take less then 10–15 minutes a day). Repeat this on Wednesday evening or day 4.

Use organic frozen vegetables if you do not have time to prepare and cook vegetables. Choose organic and choose from a wide variety from the list of vegetables in the section titled "A Special Note on what Vegetables to Buy" later in this chapter. Cascadian Farms provide good-quality organic, frozen vegetables—almost as good as fresh.

Use canned beans. Rinse and prepare according to the Tuscan bean recipe in the note on page 91 or eat straight out of the can with some olive oil, lemon, and sea salt.

You can place the beans and steamed vegetables in a container the night before with some olive oil, lemon juice, and salt, bring it to work, and heat it up.

Use wild Alaskan canned salmon as your protein source at any meal. My favorite-tasting brand is Vital Choice Seafood (www.vitalchoice.com).

Shakes are quick to prepare in the morning. They take less than 10 minutes to prepare and consume!

Ask yourself if there is there something wrong with your lifestyle that doesn't allow you to make a few simple healthy choices for one week. If you can't do it during work, then do it during a vacation. Your body will thank you!

Cooking and Preparation Suggestions

Here are a few cooking tips to make your week even simpler.

A little planning and preparation will go a long way to making your week effective and simple.

Your meals are intended to be delicious, as well as quick and simple to prepare.

Here's what to do.

Vegetables

Steam or sauté your vegetables with some fresh spices.

To steam simply:

- ✧ Put 1 cup of water in the bottom of a sauce pan.
- ✧ Purchase a steaming rack (you can get it at any grocery store for about $2) and place it over the water.
- ✧ Chop your veggies, place them in the steaming rack, cover and steam them for 4–8 minutes depending on the vegetable and your desired level of tenderness.
- ✧ Add your favorite seasonings, drizzle with extra-virgin olive oil, and add a little sea salt to taste.

You can cook almost any vegetable this way. It's easy. It's delicious. And it takes almost no time at all.

To sauté:

- ✧ Put 1 tbsp. of olive oil in the bottom of a frying pan. Turn the heat on medium high.
- ✧ Chop your veggies and drop them in.
- ✧ Sauté for 5–7 minutes for desired flavor and tenderness.
- ✧ You can also add onions, garlic, and/or mushrooms (shiitake are particularly tasty) to sautéed veggies to make them more flavorful. To do this you might want to add your onions, garlic, and mushrooms first with a little salt, sauté them, and then drop in your chopped veggies.

Fish and Chicken

Fish and chicken are very simple. Just grill, broil, or sauté your fish or chicken; season with olive oil, lemon juice, rosemary, garlic, ginger, or cilantro. Here's how.

To broil:

- ◈ Sprinkle some sea salt and whatever other seasoning you choose on your fish or chicken, and place it under the broiler.
- ◈ Fish will probably take around 7–10 minutes. Just watch it until the fish or chicken is tender and white throughout. Chicken will take longer, perhaps up to 15 minutes. You will know it's done when you press the chicken with your finger and it's relatively firm.

To grill:

- ◈ Simply season your fish or chicken and put it down on the grill. That's it. The same cooking times above apply. Turn once halfway through cooking.

To sauté:

- ◈ Place 1 tbsp. of olive oil in the bottom of a frying pan. Turn the heat on medium high.
- ◈ Heat up your oil first. Then place your seasoned fish or chicken in the pan.
- ◈ Turn regularly to avoid browning the fish or chicken too much on one side. This will be particularly important for chicken. Fish should be turned only once.
- ◈ Follow the instructions for time above.
- ◈ As with the instructions for sautéing vegetables, you could add onions, garlic, mushrooms, or even vege-

tables to this dish to change it up and make it interesting.

You can season your fish or chicken once it is done cooking with sea salt and 1 tsp. to 1 tbsp. of extra-virgin olive oil and lemon juice if you choose. (Note you probably won't add more extra-virgin olive oil if you sauté.)

Legumes

Heat up canned beans (I prefer the small white canellini or navy beans) with 1–2 tbsp. of extra-virgin olive oil, some fresh rosemary, and sea salt. Add sautéed, chopped vegetables to the beans. Be creative.

Tofu

Follow the same guidelines for fish or chicken or simply add tofu to your steamed or sautéed vegetables.

Cooking Rice

To cook brown rice boil 4 cups of filtered water, rinse 2 cups of dried brown rice, put it in the water with 1 tbsp. of olive oil and ½ tsp. of sea salt, cover, and leave covered. Bring this to a boil. Then reduce it to a simmer. Continue simmering on the lowest heat for 45 minutes. Do not stir. Optional: add 1 tsp. of turmeric or 2 round ¼-inch slices of ginger to the water when cooking. These are powerful anti-inflammatories.

Spice Up Your Food

Remember to add spices to your cooking. Place some slices of ginger in the cooked brown rice or add 1–2 tsp. of turmeric for delicious yellow, Indian-style rice. Add fresh rosemary, chopped fresh cilantro, or fresh crushed garlic to your vegetables.

Then serve. That's all there is to it.

Combine that with the UltraShake and the UltraBroth (as recommended above), and it's all you will need to reboot your metabolism and feel fantastic.

That's it. No fancy recipes, no long preparation times. Just simple, real, whole, allergen-free foods.

Getting everything ready before the week starts will make your week go smoothly and help you achieve maximum results. I can't emphasize enough the benefits of being prepared, having all your ingredients ready, and spending a little time up front preparing and cooking what you need for the week.

Let's review these simple cooking and preparation suggestions:

⬧ Pick simple preparation methods such as sautéing, grilling, or broiling for fish and chicken.

⬧ Mix up the flavors of your fish and chicken by changing your cooking methods and adding in various spices from the list I gave you above. This will help you keep from getting tired of eating the same thing every day.

⬧ Steam the vegetables, or lightly sauté in olive oil with garlic and ginger and a little bit of salt.

⬧ Cook 2 cups of brown rice at once and keep it in a tightly sealed container in the fridge. Heat it up just before eating.

⬧ Precut or chop a few days worth of vegetables and keep them in sealed glass containers or Ziploc baggies so you can steam or sauté them when you're ready.

⬧ Soak nuts overnight in water to make them easier to blend, and store them in your fridge to have them ready for your UltraShake.

Helpful Tips During the Program

- ✧ Try to start on a Sunday, doing the preparation on a Saturday, to give yourself time to acclimatize to the program. This is very important.
- ✧ Try to eat or drink something every 1–2 hours during the day to maintain energy and well-being.
- ✧ The UltraBroth can be taken anytime you feel weak or hungry.
- ✧ You may feel foggy or fatigued on the first day or two; this should clear up quickly.
- ✧ If you feel tired, rest or take a nap
- ✧ Make sure you are drinking plenty of water—6–8 glasses a day.
- ✧ Make sure you are having at least one bowel movement a day; otherwise you may feel more toxic, with feelings of fatigue, sluggishness, brain fog, headaches, bloating, and more.

If you would like more structured, step-by-step instructions on how to prepare your food, I have included some of my favorite recipes in the downloadable guide at www.ultrasimplediet.com/guide.

Additional Recipes

Although I didn't have enough room in this book to include full-blown recipes, I've included several very simple ones that follow the guidelines above that you can download in the companion guide by going to www.ultrasimplediet.com/guide.

In addition, once you join the community, you can exchange recipe ideas with other people who are on the program, thus providing even more options. To register for the community, please be sure to visit www.ultrasimplediet.com/join.

Following the Program Day by Day

In chapters 9–15 I have laid these steps out in an easy to follow day-by-day planner. There you will find detailed checklists that will help you keep track of what you have done each day on the program. Simply check off each step as you go, and make your 7-day program even easier.

In those chapters you will also find tips that will make the program more interesting, more fun, and more powerful. Incorporate those tips as you wish. You will find they are a wonderful way to feel *even better* during your program.

I have also included journaling exercises that will help you reflect on your progress, if you choose to make this a part of your program.

To make your 7 days ultrasimple, follow that planner as closely as you can. You will find it an invigorating way to improve your health and lose weight.

The UltraBroth Recipe

On this program, I suggest you drink 3–4 cups of vegetable broth per day. The broth is a wonderful, filling snack that will also provide you with many healing nutrients and alkalinize your system, making it easier to detoxify, lose weight, and feel great.

Our modern diet is an acid-producing diet—including sugar, excess animal protein, and processed foods. This acid-forming diet creates a toxic cellular environment. Our cells function optimally in a slightly alkaline environment.

Many modern diseases are related to excess acidity in the body. Detoxification can only happen if we reduce the acidity in our bodies. The UltraBroth is a simple way to alkalinize your body and can be enjoyed during the 7-day program and beyond.

The following recipe can be varied according to taste.
For every three quarts of water add:

  1 large chopped onion
  2 sliced carrots
  1 cup of daikon or white radish root and tops (ideal, but
    optional)
  1 cup of winter squash cut into large cubes
  1 cup of root vegetables: turnips, parsnips, and rutabagas for
    sweetness
  2 cups of chopped greens: kale, parsley, beet greens, collard
    greens, chard, dandelion, cilantro, or other greens
  2 celery stalks
  ½ cup of seaweed: nori, dulse, wakame, kelp, or kombu
  ½ cup of cabbage
  4½-inch slices of fresh ginger
  2 cloves of whole garlic (not chopped or crushed)
  Sea salt to taste
  If available, you can add 1 cup of fresh or dried shiitake or
    maitake mushrooms. (These have powerful immune-boosting
    properties.)

Add all the ingredients at once and place on a **low** boil for approximately 60 minutes. It may take a little longer. Simply continue to boil to taste.

Cool, strain (throw out the cooked vegetables), and store in a large, tightly sealed glass container in the fridge.

Simply heat gently and drink at least 3–4 cups a day.

Makes approximately 8 cups or 2 quarts.

A Few Notes about the Broth

When you are done making the broth, you may discard the vegetables as they are not intended to be eaten (but make sure you keep the broth!).

Feel free to mix, match, and vary the vegetables to create your own variation of the broth.

You need to wash the vegetables well, and scrub the root vegetables with a vegetable brush, but you don't need to peel them. Cut them into large chunks so you can fit them in the pot.

For those who just can't make the broth, you can substitute low-sodium, organic vegetable broth from Pacific Foods or Imagine Foods, but it is a second best to fresh broth.

The UltraShake Recipe

This shake provides essential protein for detoxification, omega-3 fatty acids from flax oil, fiber for healthy digestion, increased elimination from flaxseeds, and anti-oxidants and phytonutrients from the berries and fruit.

It will sustain you, even out your blood sugar, and help you control your appetite throughout the day.

You may alter the shake recipe to your taste preference or may even use one of the alternative breakfast recipes available in the downloadable guide at www.ultrasimplediet.com/guide instead. These recipes will incorporate most of the healing ingredients in the shake. However, the shake is designed to be quick, easy, and contain powerful healing ingredients to help you with inflammation and detoxification.

Version 1: Using Rice Protein

This shake is the easiest to make and digest and quite satisfying.

    2 scoops of rice protein powder (The average is 2 scoops, but
       you should follow the directions for the serving sizes of the
       product you pick.)
    1 tbsp. of organic combination flax and borage oil
    2 tbsp. of ground flaxseeds

Ice (made from filtered water), if desired

6–8 ounces of filtered water to desired consistency (some like
  thicker drinks, some thinner)

½ cup of frozen or fresh, noncitrus organic fruit such as
  cherries, blueberries, raspberries, strawberries, peaches,
  pears, or frozen bananas

Optional: add 1 tbsp. of nut butter (almond, macadamia,
  pecan) or ¼ cup of nuts soaked overnight such as almonds,
  walnuts, pecans, or any combination of these

For Better Tasting Shakes: Adding frozen cherries, ½ a frozen banana, and nut butters provides the best-tasting shakes.

Special Note on Rice Protein: I prefer detoxifying hypoaller-
genic rice protein. While it can be expensive, it replaces meals
and facilitates your detoxifying and weight loss during the
week.

Note: Use the flax seeds in up to two shakes a day, no more.

Version 2: Fruit and Nut Smoothie

If you don't want to use rice protein (which needs to be purchased) you can simply use silken tofu. This is a nice creamy,
shake made from real food.

¼ cup of silken drained tofu

½ cup of plain, unsweetened, gluten-free soy milk (such as Silk)

1 tbsp. of organic, combination flax and borage oil

2 tbsp. of ground flaxseeds

½ cup of fresh or frozen, noncitrus organic fruit such as
  cherries, blueberries, raspberries, strawberries, peaches,
  pears, or frozen bananas

Optional: add 1 tbsp. of nut butter (almond, macadamia,
  pecan) or ¼ cup of nuts soaked overnight such as almonds,
  walnuts, pecans, or any combination of these

Ice (made from filtered water), if desired

2–4 ounces of filtered water to desired consistency, (some like
  thicker drinks, some thinner)

For Better Tasting Shakes: Adding frozen cherries, ½ a frozen banana, and nut butters provides the best tasting shakes.

Note: Use the flax seeds in up to two shakes a day, no more.

Version 3: Nut Smoothie

This shake is designed to be soy-free. It requires no extra purchase of powder, and can be made from easily accessible ingredients.

> ½ cup of plain, unsweetened, gluten-free almond or hazelnut milk
> 1–2 tbsp. of nut butter (almond, macadamia, pecan) or ¼ cup of nuts soaked overnight such as almonds, walnuts, pecans, or any combination of these
> 1 tbsp. organic, combination flax and borage oil
> 2 tbsp. ground flaxseeds
> ½ cup of fresh or frozen, noncitrus organic fruit such as cherries, blueberries, raspberries, strawberries, peaches, pears, or frozen bananas
> Ice (made from filtered water), if desired
> 2–4 ounces of filtered water to desired consistency, (some like thicker drinks, some thinner)

For Better Tasting Shakes: Adding frozen cherries, ½ a frozen banana, and nut butters provides the best tasting shakes.

Note: Use the flax seeds in up to two shakes a day, no more.

The UltraBath

The UltraBath is a key component of the program. It provides many powerful benefits in one easy, 20-minute solution every day. This may not sound important, but the UltraBath has been one of the most favorite features of those who have experienced the program.

The benefits of the UltraBath include:

- ✧ Relaxation of your nervous system and lowering of cortisol through the use of lavender oil, which promotes weight loss and lowers inflammation.
- ✧ Enhancement of detoxification through the effects of the magnesium and sulfur in the Epsom salts.
- ✧ Enhanced sleep through the effects of the hot bath and magnesium.
- ✧ Alkalinization of your body through the use of baking soda (sodium bicarbonate), which promotes an ideal pH for healing, detoxification, and optimal cellular function.
- ✧ Increased circulation and increased heart rate, which serves as a form of passive exercise.
- ✧ Lowered blood pressure and blood sugar levels.
- ✧ Increased heart rate variability, a sign of a healthy nervous system and reduced stress.
- ✧ Increased sweating and elimination of toxins.

Add 2 cups of Epsom salts, 1 cup of baking soda, and 10 drops of lavender oil to bathwater as hot as you can tolerate.

Take a 20-minute UltraBath just before bed every night.

For extra-powerful detoxification wrap yourself in towels immediately after the bath, get in bed under the covers and sweat more for 20 minutes, then remove the towels and go to sleep. You can go directly to sleep without rinsing off after the bath.

You can also take a sauna or steam bath for up to 30 minutes per day if it is available to you.

Shopping List

The quantities on this checklist should take care of all your needs for one week on the program.

All ingredients should be organic if possible.

You can download this shopping list by going to www.ultrasimplediet.com/guide and downloading *The UltraSimple Companion Guide.* That way it will be easy to print out and take to the store with you.

✓	Quantity	Type of Food
		Protein You can choose from any combination of the following. Amounts will vary depending on how much of each you choose to eat
	1¾–2¾ pounds of fish or chicken combined	Fish—small, non-predatory species such as ✦ Sardines ✦ Herring ✦ Wild salmon ✦ Black cod ✦ Sable fish ✦ Sole ✦ Cod
		Boneless, skinless, chicken breast (preferably organic)
	3 pounds	Tofu
	4 cans	Canned beans. Choose from the following: ✦ Cannellini beans ✦ Navy beans ✦ Chick peas
		Vegetables You will need LOTS of these!
	½–2 pounds per meal depending on your appetite	Choose a variety from each category identified in "A Special Note on What Vegetables to Buy" below. You should have enough to steam 2 cups each for lunch and dinner, and to make the UltraBroth (see recipe above). You can eat as many vegetables as you like. Buy enough so you're not hungry.

✓	Quantity	Type of Food
		Whole Grains
	6 cups	Brown rice, long or short grain
		Oil
	1 liter	Extra-virgin olive oil
		Beverages
	Approximately 7 gallons, or enough for 8–10 glasses per day	Filtered or distilled water or purchase a reverse osmosis or Brita filter to purify your water
	1 box of tea or 8 ounces of loose leaf	Green tea, preferably organic, decaf or caffeinated
		Spices These spices have powerful anti-inflammatory and detoxifying properties, which is why I recommend them for this program. You can use them to your personal tastes.
	1 large root (4 ounces)	Fresh ginger
	2 heads (or you can purchase prepeeled cloves for convenience)	Whole garlic cloves
	8–12	Lemons (Though these aren't a spice, you can still use them to spice up your food. But don't forget they are an important part of the program for other reasons as well.)
	1 small bottle	Turmeric (the yellow spice found in curry—add 1–2 teaspoons to the water you cook your rice in)
	1 bunch	Rosemary (fresh is best)
	1–2 bunches	Cilantro (also known as coriander—fresh is best)

✓	Quantity	Type of Food
	1–2 peppers goes a long way!	Chili peppers (fresh is best)
	1 bottle	Whole black peppercorns for the pepper mill
	1 bottle	Sea salt*
		UltraShake Version 1
	1 large bottle	Rice protein powder
	4–6 cups or 2–3 packages of Cascadian Farms organic fruit	Fresh or frozen noncitrus (i.e., no oranges, grapefruit, or tangerines) fruit such as cherries, blueberries, blackberries, or strawberries. (This will also be enough to eat for dessert twice a week.)
	1 15-ounce package or the equivalent in whole, bulk flax seed.	Ground flaxseeds. Fiproflax is the freshest organic ground flax on the market. Be sure to keep it refrigerated. You can buy flaxseeds already ground, or you can buy them whole and grind them yourself in a coffee grinder.
	1 large bottle	Combination flax and borage oil, organic, high lignan. Barlean's or Spectrum are the best brands.
	2 cups	**Optional:** Nuts and seeds: almonds, walnuts, pecans, macadamia nuts, and pumpkin seeds
	1 jar	Nut butter (almond, macadamia, or pecan)
		UltraShake Version 2
	7 cups	Silken tofu (Note: This amount is in addition to the amounts of tofu recommended for your meals above.)

* Use only sea salt during the program. Table salt is mined from underground salt deposits and includes a small portion of calcium silicate, an anti-caking agent added to prevent clumping. Because of its fine grain a single teaspoon of table salt contains more salt than a tablespoon of kosher or sea salt.

Sea salt is harvested from evaporated seawater and receives little or no processing. It contains nearly 50 minerals that support our health.

✓	Quantity	Type of Food
	14 cups	Unsweetened, gluten-free soy milk (such as Silk)
	4–6 cups or 2–3 packages of Cascadian Farms organic fruit	Fresh or frozen noncitrus (i.e., no oranges, grapefruit, or tangerines) fruit such as cherries, blueberries, blackberries, or strawberries. (This will also be enough to eat for dessert twice a week.)
	1 15-ounce package or the equivalent in whole, bulk flax seed.	Ground flaxseeds. Fiproflax is the freshest organic ground flax on the market. Be sure to keep it refrigerated. You can buy flaxseeds already ground, or you can buy them whole and grind them yourself in a coffee grinder.
	1 12-ounce bottle	Combination flax and borage oil, organic, high lignan. Barlean's or Spectrum are the best brands.
	2 cups	**Optional:** Nuts and seeds: almonds, walnuts, pecans, macadamia nuts, and pumpkin seeds
	1 jar	Nut butter (almond, macadamia, or pecan)
	UltraShake Version 3	
	14 cups	Plain, unsweetened almond or hazelnut milk
	2 cups	Nuts and seeds: almonds, walnuts, pecans, macadamia nuts and pumpkin seeds
	1 jar	Nut butter (almond, macadamia, or pecan)
	4–6 cups or 2–3 packages of Cascadian Farms organic fruit	Fresh or frozen noncitrus (i.e., no oranges, grapefruit, or tangerines) fruit such as cherries, blueberries, blackberries, or strawberries. (This will also be enough to eat for dessert twice a week.)
	1 12-ounce bottle	Combination flax and borage oil, organic, high lignan. Barlean's or Spectrum are the best brands.

✓	Quantity	Type of Food
	1 15-ounce package or the equivalent in whole, bulk flax seed.	Ground flaxseeds. Fiproflax is the freshest organic ground flax on the market. Be sure to keep it refrigerated. You can buy flaxseeds already ground, or you can buy them whole and grind them yourself in a coffee grinder
	UltraBroth Needs to be multiplied x 3–4 batches depending how much broth you consume per day. Note that the following amounts are in addition to recommendations above.	
	1 large	Onion
	2	Carrots
	1 cup	Daikon or white radish root and tops (ideal, but optional)
	1 cup	Winter squash
	1 cup	Root vegetables: turnips, parsnips, and rutabagas for sweetness
	2 cups or 1 bunch	Greens: kale, parsley, beet greens, collard greens, chard, dandelion, cilantro and/or other greens
	2 stalks	Celery
	½ cup	Seaweed: nori, dulse, wakame, kelp, or kombu*
	½ cup	Cabbage
	4½-inch slices	Fresh ginger root
	2 cloves	Whole garlic (not chopped or crushed)
	1 cup	Fresh or dried shiitake or maitake mushrooms, if available. (These have powerful immune-boosting properties.)
	UltraBath Note: Amounts may vary depending on what your local store sells.	

* Seaweed is a new food for most people. It is purchased dry in packages and simply needs to be broken off, measured, and thrown in the broth.

✓	Quantity	Type of Food
	1 large box or 2 liters	Baking Soda
	4–6 ½-gallon containers	Epsom Salts
	1 small bottle	Lavender Essential Oil
		If You are Constipated Use these products as directed in Chapter 5
	1 bottle	Magnesium citrate capsules or tablets
	1 bottle of powder or capsules	Buffered ascorbic acid (vitamin C)
	1 bottle	Herbal laxative
	1 bottle	Magnesium citrate liquid.
	1–2 of each	Dulcolax or Bisacodyl Suppository or Fleet Enema

A Special Note on What Vegetables to Buy

During the program, you may choose from the following vegetables at lunch or dinner. These veggies maximize phytonutrient (powerful disease-fighting chemicals found in colorful plant foods) intake, and include powerful detoxifying and anti-inflammatory compounds.

Choose vegetables from all of the categories. Use vegetables you like already, but also experiment and try something new!

I encourage you to eat primarily cooked vegetables (either steamed or sautéed) during the program, because they are easier to digest. While you may still enjoy salads or raw vegetables, keep them to a minimum. Use extra-virgin olive oil, lemon juice, and salt and pepper for dressing.

Vegetables

Allium vegetables: Garlic, onions, leeks, and shallots

Cruciferous vegetables: Broccoli, cabbage, kale, collard greens, kohlrabi, Brussels sprouts, bok choy, and Chinese broccoli

Dark blue, purple, or red fruits and vegetables: Cherries, blueberries, blackberries, beets, red onions, purple grapes, red cabbage, and radicchio*

Dark green, leafy vegetables: Spinach, watercress, arugula, collard greens, kale, cabbage, Brussels sprouts, and loose-leaf lettuce (not iceberg lettuce)

Red and yellow vegetables: Chili peppers, sweet potatoes (a different plant family than regular potatoes), winter squash (like acorn, butternut, buttercup, or kabocha squash), and carrots

Special detoxifying vegetables: Artichokes or artichoke hearts, asparagus, beets, celery, and dandelion greens

Sea vegetables: Nori, kelp, dulse, kombu, hijiki, arame, and wakame

Root vegetables for broth: Sweet potatoes, rutabagas, turnips, parsnips, and carrots

----

Summary

✧ During the program, you will avoid sugar, refined carbohydrates, trans fats, alcohol, caffeine, pro-

----

* Please use the berries only in the shake and ½ cup as a treat a few days during the diet. They are NOT to be eaten in unlimited quantities.

cessed and junk foods, and all of the most common food allergens.

✧ You will enjoy fresh, whole, organic, detoxifying, and anti-inflammatory foods such as vegetables, fruit, fish, chicken, tofu, beans, nuts, and seeds.

✧ You can even follow the program if you are extremely busy by making a few simple changes in the program.

✧ The UltraShake, the UltraBroth, and the UltraBath all help support you through the powerful detoxifying and anti-inflammatory UltraSimple Diet.

What's Next

For a deeper experience, you can try the enhanced program explained in the next chapter.

CHAPTER 8

The Enhanced UltraSimple Diet

*"6 pounds lost this week, plus the 5 pounds
the week before in the pre-diet . . ."*

*I have an active family (3 school-age children). I work full-
time. I am in graduate school and after starting school, I discovered I am a "stress eater." After 7 months I had gained 30
pounds on an already overweight frame . . . When I read The
UltraSimple Diet and saw there was an "enhanced" version
for stress relief, I decided it was an answer to my prayer! And it
has been! I was stunned! After the first day I felt so much better,
not bloated and heavy . . . The broth is really good and my
children comment on how fresh the kitchen smells when I'm
cooking up a pot! . . . 6 pounds lost this week, plus the 5 pounds
the week before in the pre-diet, I'm excited! . . . I can see a difference and that feels great! It is the motivation I needed. I recommend this plan!*

Helen Meeks
Blakely, GA

For more success stories, go to www.ultrasimplediet.com/success.

In this chapter you will learn:

  ✧ The program for The Enhanced UltraSimple Diet
  ✧ How to use supplements, exercise, and relaxation
    techniques to boost your results

Following the enhanced program adds another important dimension to your experience, and provides you a foundation for ongoing health, wellness, and weight loss. It adds these important elements:

- ✧ Supplements
- ✧ Exercise
- ✧ Relaxation and Stress Reduction

Here is the overview of the enhanced program.

Optional Daily Sample Schedule

- ✧ Wake up 90–120 minutes before you need to leave the house.

Upon Waking

- ✧ 2 tbsp. organic extra-virgin olive oil mixed with the juice of ½ of an organic lemon—drink down to help flush the toxins from your bile and liver into your gut to be excreted*
- ✧ 1 tsp. buffered ascorbic acid (vitamin C) powder in 8 ounces of water or 2–3 1000-mg capsules of buffered ascorbic acid (vitamin C) powder**

---

* Your liver eliminates toxins via the bile. Drinking olive oil and lemon juice stimulates the production of bile and the excretion of toxins from your liver into your gut, where they can be eliminated.

This can be taken at any time of the day but should be taken on an empty stomach. The ideal times are upon waking, mid-morning, afternoon, or before bed.

** I suggest you take specific supplements at certain times of the day for a reason.

Morning Ritual

- ❖ 20–60 minutes yoga
- ❖ 20 minutes journaling

Breakfast (7-9 a.m.)

- ❖ Lemon juice (from ½ lemon) and hot water
- ❖ 1 cup of decaf or caffeinated green tea, steeped in hot water for 5 minutes (You may also have the green tea later in the day. Limit your intake to 2 cups a day.)
- ❖ 2 capsules probiotics before eating
- ❖ 2 capsules of liver supportive herbs and nutrients before eating
- ❖ UltraShake
- ❖ If no bowel movement by 10 in the morning, take 2 capsules or tablets of an herbal laxative*

Morning Snack (10-11 a.m.)

- ❖ 1 cup UltraBroth
- ❖ Another UltraShake without fiber or combination flax and borage oil (if you are hungry)

Lunch (12-1 p.m.)

- ❖ 2 tablets magnesium citrate with the meal (average capsule or tablet is 100–150 mg)

* More information about how to take herbal laxatives can be found in chapter 5. You will also find more specific recommendations about the types of laxatives you might consider in *The UltraSimple Companion Guide*. See www.ultrasimplediet.com/guide for more details.

✧ 2 cups or more of steamed or lightly sautéed veggies
  (You should eat enough to feel gently satisfied.)
✧ ½ cup cooked brown rice
✧ ½ cup fruit or berries for dessert (Either here or
  at dinner, not both, and only 1–2 times during the
  7-day program.)
✧ UltraShake (optional)

Afternoon Snack (2–3 p.m.)

✧ 1 cup UltraBroth
✧ UltraShake (if you are hungry)

Afternoon rest if possible for 30 minutes, or leisurely walk

Before Dinner

✧ 30-minute walk or aerobic exercise
✧ Sauna or steam at least 3 times a week if possible
✧ 20 minutes yoga

Dinner (5–7 p.m.)

✧ 2 capsules of probiotics before eating
✧ 2 capsules of liver detox supportive herbs and nutrients before eating
✧ 2 cups or more of steamed or lightly sautéed veggies
  (You should eat enough to feel gently satisfied.)
✧ ½ cup of brown rice
✧ 4–6 ounces of fish or chicken or tofu or beans
✧ 1 cup UltraBroth

Bedtime or Evening Ritual

✧ 20 minutes restorative yoga
✧ 20 minutes journaling (if desired)

✦ 3 capsules of herbal laxative (if no bowel movement
   that day)

✦ 2 capsules or tablets of magnesium citrate

✦ 20-minute UltraBath

This helps them interact with your body in the most effective way possible.

However, if you already have a routine established for taking supplements and you wish to take the supplements on the enhanced program in conjunction with your other supplements you may do that. It won't cause any problems as regards the program.

Another note: If you forget to take your supplements and remember later in the day, go ahead and take them. It's better to get them in at some point than not to take them at all.

Supplements

While it is not necessary to take any supplements during the basic program, they can be a powerful addition to your health program.

Those on the basic program need not take ANY supplements and can still receive about 80 percent of the benefits from the program. For those who want to get that extra 20 percent benefit that supplements, exercise, and working on the emotional and spiritual side of their transformation may offer, I recommend the enhanced program.

For that reason, the enhanced program includes recommendations for specific supplements to take during the one-week program.

Why Supplements Are So Important

Based on decades of research and a new understanding of the role of vitamins, minerals, and omega-3 fats in health, I recommend that everyone be on a basic supplement regimen to prevent disease and promote health on an ongoing basis, regardless of whether you are doing the program in this book or not. You should plan on getting these supplements and making them a part of your life.

IMPORTANT: You do not NEED to do it during the basic or enhanced plans, but you should do it at some point.

For the long term, after you are finished with the program, I recommend everyone take the following basic supplements. These can be started any time before, during, or after the program. The most important thing is to take them!

IMPORTANT: Please do not confuse this as being in addition to the supplements for the enhanced program; rather, these are recommended for life-long vitality AFTER you've finished the program.

Basic supplements

✦ A high quality multivitamin and mineral supplement
✦ High quality omega-3 fats—fish oil capsules or liquid
✦ Calcium, magnesium, and vitamin D
✦ Probiotics—healthy bacteria for the gut that promote healthy digestion and reduce inflammation and allergy

You can find more details on choosing high-quality products as well as the recommended dosages for each one in the downloadable *UltraSimple Companion Guide* which you can get at www.ultrasimplediet.com/guide.

Why Do We Need Supplements Anyway?

The typical American's diet is horribly deficient in vitamins, minerals, and other nutrients. In fact, 92 percent of Americans don't get the minimum daily required level of one or more nutrients.

Why are these nutrients so important you may ask?

Vitamins and minerals are the essential chemical helpers that make all the chemical reactions in your body run smoothly. Without them, your biochemistry grinds to a halt. This manifests itself as many common symptoms and diseases that are unrecognized by most physicians.

If you have scurvy, everybody knows you need vitamin C. But what about more mild vitamin or mineral deficiencies? For example, if you are magnesium deficient you may experience constipation, muscle cramps, painful menstrual periods, anxiety, palpitations, insomnia, and headaches.

If you are deficient in folate or B-12 you can become depressed, have memory problems, and even suffer from symptoms that mimic multiple sclerosis. And you won't be able to prevent cancer, heart disease, or dementia.

If you are deficient in omega-3 fats (which more than 90 percent of Americans are) you may have dry, pasty skin, weak nails, lackluster hair, depression, dry mouth, and you are at much higher risk for weight gain, diabetes, heart attacks, strokes, dementia, and cancer.

There are dozens of vitamins and minerals we require for health. Without enough of them on a daily basis, our bodies cannot function optimally.

Unless you are eating foods picked straight from your organic garden (not grown in nutrient-depleted soils or stored and transported thousands of miles), you are eating nutrient-depleted foods.

That's why it is so important to take the basic supplement program I recommend, every day, for the rest of your life.

You can start it after the program, but be sure to start it.

The additional supplements for the enhanced program are designed to be used DURING the 7-day program and may help with detoxification, elimination, reducing inflammation, and promoting weight loss and healing. The basic supplements (a multivitamin, fish oil, calcium, magnesium, and vitamin D) are not needed during the enhanced program.

The basic supplements, the enhanced supplements, and other supplements I discuss in my book *UltraMetabolism: The Simple Plan for Automatic Weight Loss,* contain critical nutrients that may help you turn on your "ultrametabolism," which is your body's ability to function at top performance.

That's why I strongly recommend you take the essential basic supplements every day. Adding probiotics to support your digestive health and reduce inflammation and food allergies can be another important addition to your program.

You should take the basic supplement package whether or not you are on a diet. These are supplements you need for your continued health. Of course, you don't HAVE to, but I STRONGLY recommend it.

The Enhanced UltraSimple Supplements

These are the supplements to take during the enhanced version of the program.

In the downloadable *UltraSimple Companion Guide* I've included more information on the types of supplements that I give to my patients in my private medical practice, precise details for the type of ingredients you should look for and how to select high-quality brands, and a timing checklist for exactly when you should take these supplements. Go to www.ultra simplediet.com/guide for more information.

Dosage	Supplement
2 capsules	Acidophilus/bifidus combination to restore healthy gut bacteria, reduce inflammation, and reduce allergies

Dosage	Supplement
1000–2000 mg one to two times a day	Buffered ascorbic acid (vitamin C) powder or capsules to enhance detoxification, reduce inflammation, and help move bowels
2–3 capsules a day	Herbal laxative (if needed) to help clear out the bowels
2 100–150 mg capsules or tablets, twice a day	Magnesium citrate to help over 300 chemical enzymes in your body and to help prevent constipation
2 scoops per shake	Rice protein–based nutritional detoxification shake (This is used as part of the UltraShake. It contains special nutrients and amino acids that promote detoxification beside just the low-allergy rice protein. This is different than a pure rice protein powder and is preferred.)
2 capsules twice a day	Liver detoxification supportive herbs and nutrients that boost all the liver detoxification pathways.

These supplements and nutrients are all available at your local health food store or can be ordered online. More information on the benefits and the details of these types of supplements can be found in *The UltraSimple Companion Guide*. You can download it by going to www.ultrasimplediet.com/guide.

While I do not endorse any particular company or product, hopefully the suggestions in the downloadable *UltraSimple Companion Guide* will help you pick high-quality products. Go to www.ultrasimple.com/guide for more details.

Each person must use his or her own discretion and knowledge of their personal health conditions when choosing supplements or other health-related products. I strongly advise you to seek the assistance of a doctor trained in nutritional medicine or nutritionist to help personalize your supplement program.

Exercise

The role of exercise in health and weight loss is clear to nearly everyone now. It must be an essential part of any long-term strategy for achieving optimal health.

However, I find that many of my patients who are overweight, toxic, and inflamed don't have the energy or ability to exercise right away.

That's fine. Once they start to heal, exercise becomes much easier.

During the enhanced program exercise can be an added bonus for those who choose it. It may help increase your circulation, facilitate elimination of toxins, help you sweat, reduce stress, and boost your metabolism.

The good news is that I recommend only gentle walking during the 7-day program. You don't want to push your body too far. This week is for healing and repair. Be gentle with yourself. Doing the simple walking I recommend can increase your energy, help your digestion, improve your sleep, and help you lose more weight.

Here is what I recommend:

- ✧ Walk daily during the week for a minimum of 30 minutes each time. Be sure you have a comfortable pair of walking shoes with ample cushioning and arch support.
- ✧ That's it! You can vary the speed and distance, walk hills or no hills, but just get out, breathe fresh air, and enjoy yourself.

Relaxation and Stress Management

Thousands of years ago, stress was our friend, and it served us well. When we were confronted with danger—like a predator that wanted to eat us—stress chemicals would quickly flood the body, enhancing our ability to either fight or flee. As soon as the danger dissipated, the stress-chemical levels would quickly drop, and so would the feelings of stress.

Today, however, we're under *constant* stress. We're bombarded by inputs from the media, cell phones, pagers, computers, e-mail, voice mail, and faxes. We're inundated with bad news, bad relationships, stressful jobs, and difficult living environments. Even worse, just *thinking about negative things—* whether they're real or not—can trigger the stress response. So understanding stress and how you can reduce it is critical to living a healthy and happy life.

How Stress Damages Your Health

The body responds to stress by releasing hormones, including one called cortisol. Cortisol levels are supposed to go up and down quickly. But when you're under chronic stress, cortisol continues to pump out. And it triggers a cascade of events.

For example, cortisol causes fat to be stored around your middle. That belly fat causes most of the "silent inflammation" that leads to diabetes, heart disease, and virtually all other chronic conditions that humans suffer from.

By decreasing mental stress and noticing the profound benefits to your nervous system, sleep habits, and digestion, you will learn about the subtle but powerful connection between psychological, spiritual, and physical toxins. When your nervous system is balanced, when you are rested, and when your digestion is working properly, you may find you have much more energy for your everyday life.

Stress, by contrast, is fatiguing. Fatigue is demoralizing. And demoralization may lead us to seek quick highs from sugar, caffeine, alcohol, and other drugs.

Reducing stress requires *active* relaxation. Most of us think relaxation is a passive "nonactivity" that requires a couch, a beer, and a TV. But stress reduction requires profound, deep relaxation, which is not something that happens automatically. You have to *actively* relax.

Here are some simple tips to relax, calm your nervous system, and reduce stress:

- ✧ Take an UltraBath
- ✧ Yoga
- ✧ Meditation
- ✧ Guided relaxation
- ✧ Biofeedback and tools for improving heart rate variability
- ✧ Splurge and get a massage or facial.
- ✧ Deep breathing
- ✧ Stop rushing. Give yourself more time.
- ✧ Spend time in a place of beauty such as the beach, a garden or the woods. Don't do anything, just observe the beauty around you.
- ✧ Cut down on TV, fluff reading, and aimless internet surfing.
- ✧ Limit exposure to news. Take a break from the world's troubles.
- ✧ Limit exposure to people who make you feel bad.

Napping

Napping is another simple addition to the enhanced program. In our culture, we have been taught "no pain, no gain." The truth is that in order to become strong and healthy, our bodies require rest. During rest, our tissues regenerate, detoxify, and heal. In addition, when our body rests, our mind also has a chance to recuperate.

If at all possible, try and take a 20- to 30-minute nap each day during your 7-day program. If taking a daily nap is simply impossible, try to make napping a part of your weekends.

Take a Media Holiday

To further rest your mind, give yourself a break from television or radio news broadcasts, newspapers, "spaced-out" television watching, and surfing the Internet. If you're not engaged in working, relaxing, self-care, and/or spending time with friends or loved ones, just let your mind rest.

See what happens when you don't fill empty spaces with chatter from TV, radio, newspapers, or magazines. During this 7-day period, restrict your media intake to nourishing, personally-meaningful books, movies, music, and other media that help you relax and support your health program.

Keep Work to a Minimum for 7 Days

In addition, try to limit your work to normal office hours. Try not to bring work home or schedule business-related social events during the 7-day period.

Instead, limit social engagements to those that are truly relaxing and fun. During your 7 days on the enhanced program, make sure you set aside time to hang out with friends and loved ones who truly support and nurture you.

At the end of the 7-day period, I feel certain that you'll feel more refreshed, rested, and peaceful and may have lost up to 10 pounds of toxic fluid and fat.

Following the Enhanced Program Day by Day

In chapters 9–15 you will find a planner that will help you follow the program day by day. There you will find detailed checklists that will help you keep track of where you are each day you are on the enhanced program. Simply check off each step as you go to make the program even simpler.

In those chapters you will also find specific tips for making the enhanced program more interesting, more fun, and more powerful. Incorporate them as you wish. You will find they are a wonderful way to feel *even better* during your program.

To make your 7 days ultrasimple, follow that planner as closely as you can. You will find it an invigorating way to improve your health and lose weight.

Summary

- ✧ The enhanced program boosts the basic plan with the addition of supplements, exercise, and relaxation and stress-management techniques.
- ✧ Supplements can boost your metabolism, as well as help you detoxify and reduce inflammation.
- ✧ Exercise can increase your circulation, improve digestion, help you sleep, and help you lose weight.
- ✧ Active relaxation is critical for the body's healing, repair, and weight-loss systems.

What's Next

The next 7 chapters provide a day-by-day, step-by-step guide for following the basic program and the enhanced program.

CHAPTER 9

Day 1 of The UltraSimple Diet

"I can feel my body warm up inside,
and I know my metabolism has kicked in
and all the bad stuff is getting burned away."

After just 7 days I lost 4.5 pounds, 1.5 inches off my waist and
2 inches off my hips. At 66 I look better. My skin is better. My body
shape is better. And I feel this calm, warm energy throughout my
day. I can feel my body warm up inside, and I know my metabo-
lism has kicked in and all the bad stuff is getting burned away.

Nancy Nelson
Seattle, WA

Read Nancy's whole story at the end of this chapter.

For more success stories, go to www.ultrasimplediet.com/success.

In the following chapters you will learn:

- ✧ How to follow the program step by step.
- ✧ Tips on diet, exercise, supplements, detoxifying, controlling inflammation, improving sleep, and reducing stress.

In the next few chapters, I will give you a simple day-by-day plan to follow that will transform your life.

In the checklists below you will find the basic program and the enhanced program combined in one daily schedule. Instructions for the basic program are in **bold.** Extra instructions for the enhanced program are in plain type.

If you choose to do the basic plan, go down the list and check off the actions items that are listed in bold as you complete each one of them and ignore the ones that are in plain type. If you have chosen to do the enhanced program, simply do everything on the list—the items in bold as well as the ones in plain type.

Today will be a new experience. You may feel changes to your body. The first day can be a day of readjustment from a toxic life. You might feel a bit more fatigued, and your digestion may be getting used to the new foods. You might feel a few leftover cravings. It can be an exciting and also scary day where you change so much about your diet and your life. Stay with it and you should come out the other side feeling thinner, happier, and healthier.

Checklist for Day 1

If you don't want to write in your book, I have reprinted this checklist in the downloadable *UltraSimple Companion Guide* at www.ultrasimplediet.com/guide.

Action Items for Day 1 on the Program

☐   Wake up 90–120 minutes before you need to leave the house.

Upon Waking

☐   2 tbsp. organic, extra-virgin olive oil mixed with the juice of ½ of an organic lemon—drink down to help flush the toxins from your bile and liver into your gut to be excreted

☐ 1 tsp. buffered ascorbic acid (vitamin C) powder in
  8 ounces of water or 2–3 1000-mg capsules of buffered
  ascorbic acid (vitamin C)

Morning Ritual

☐ 20–60 minutes yoga

☐ **20 minutes journaling (You can do this by printing
  the journal in the downloadable guide at www.ultra
  simplediet.com/guide or in the online version of
  the community at www.ultrasimplediet.com/join.)**

Breakfast (7–9 a.m.)

☐ **Lemon juice (from ½ lemon) and hot water**

☐ **1 cup of green tea, steeped in hot water for 5 minutes
  (You may also have the green tea later in the day. Limit
  your intake to 2 cups a day.)**

☐ 2 capsules of probiotics before eating

☐ 2 capsules of liver supportive herbs and nutrients before
  eating

☐ **UltraShake**

☐ **If no bowel movement by 10 a.m., take herbal laxative
  (2–3 capsules). If no bowel movement in 6 hours, follow
  the steps for overcoming constipation in chapter 5.**

Morning Snack (10–11 a.m.)

☐ **1 cup UltraBroth**

☐ **Another UltraShake without flaxseeds or combination
  flax and borage oil (if you are hungry)**

Lunch (12–1 p.m.)

☐ 2 capsules or tablets of magnesium citrate with the meal
  (average capsule or tablet is 100–150 mg)

☐ **2 cups or more of steamed or lightly sautéed veggies
  (You should eat enough to feel gently satisfied.)**

☐ **½ cup cooked brown rice**

☐ ½ cup fruit or berries for dessert (Either here or at dinner, not both, and only 1–2 times during the 7-day program.)

☐ UltraShake (optional)

Afternoon Snack (2–3 p.m.)

☐ 1 cup UltraBroth

☐ UltraShake (if you are hungry)

☐ Afternoon rest if possible for 30 minutes, or leisurely walk

Before Dinner

☐ 30-minute walk or aerobic exercise

☐ Sauna or steam at least 3 times a week if possible

☐ 20 minutes yoga

Dinner (5–7 p.m.)

☐ 2 capsules of probiotics before eating

☐ 2 capsules of liver detox supportive herbs and nutrients before eating

☐ 2 cups or more of steamed or lightly sautéed veggies (You should eat enough to feel gently satisfied.)

☐ ½ cup of brown rice

☐ 4–6 ounces of fish or chicken breast or 1 cup of legumes or tofu

☐ 1 cup UltraBroth

Bedtime or Evening Ritual

☐ 20 minutes restorative yoga

☐ 20 minutes journaling (if desired)

☐ 2–3 capsules of herbal laxative (if no bowel movement that day)

☐ 2 capsules of magnesium citrate

☐   **20-minute UltraBath**

☐   **Interact with others, share tips, recipes and other advice in the UltraSimple community at www.ultrasimplediet.com/join.**

* You can eat the lunch menu at dinner or the dinner menu at lunch, whatever is most convenient for you. Remember, if you prepare your food the night before, you can take it with you to work and just heat it up.

Journaling Exercises for Day 1

I've included a special section in the downloadable guide at www.ultrasimplediet.com/guide where you can keep track of your daily journaling activity. Print out the guide so you have an easy place to record your thoughts. Or, you can record them online by going to the special community at www.ultrasimplediet.com/join.

In the Morning

Do this journaling exercise in the morning on the **first day** of the program:

✧ What can I do today to truly take care of my body?

✧ What can I do today to truly take care of my spirit?

✧ What toxic food/idea/behavior can I do without today?

✧ How do I feel today, physically? Do I feel tired? Bloated? Stiff? What else do I notice about my physical state today?

✧ How do I feel today, emotionally and spiritually? Do I feel stuck? Fearful? Confused? Angry? Disconnected? Why?

✧ What else do I notice about my emotional and spiritual state that is noteworthy?

In the Evening

Do this exercise in the evening on the **first day** of the program.

- ✧ What worked for me today?
- ✧ What can I improve on tomorrow?
- ✧ What symptoms improved today?
- ✧ What did I notice about how I am feeling?
- ✧ What did I learn today on the program that I can carry with me into the rest of my life?

UltraSimple Tip of the Day

Food Tip: **Phytonutrients**

Healing chemicals in foods may in the end be more important than the protein, fat, carbohydrates, vitamins, and minerals they contain. Research has identified a whole class of compounds called phytonutrients or phytochemicals in plants that have enormous beneficial impact on our health, and their absence may lead to chronic illness.

To maximize the benefit of these healing foods, choose from the incredibly rich variety of colorful fruits and vegetables that are available. Think color! Try something different!

For more tips on boosting your metabolism with the latest science, download *The UltraSimple Companion Guide* at www.ultrasimplediet.com/guide.

An UltraSimple Case Study

I'm 66, and I was starting to get that old-lady figure. You know the one where your chest sinks down into your big round stomach? I think women my age look at themselves and just accept it. But I can't. I won't accept it.

I hoped that detoxifying would improve the bloating around my midsection. And it did!

I lost 4.5 pounds, 1.5 inches off my waist, and 2 inches off my hips in 7 days!

I started to notice the change the first day of the program. My hips and stomach started shrinking, and by the end of the week, the bloating disappeared completely. The best part is that it seems to be gone for good! It's been months, and I still haven't gained the weight back.

I look better too. My skin is better. My body shape is better. And I feel this calm, warm energy throughout my day. I can feel my body warm up inside, and I know my metabolism has kicked in and all the bad stuff is getting burned away.

People tell me I look fantastic, and ask what I'm doing. They say, "You've totally changed. Your face has changed." One woman even told me I was stunning! I have never had that word used with me before . . .

I say, "It's all because of the UltraSimple program."

Nancy Nelson
Seattle, WA

Here are Nancy's measurements before and after the program.

Measurements	Before	After	Improvement
Weight (in pounds)	159.5	155	4.5
Waist (in inches)	34.5	33	1.5
Hips (in inches)	43	41	2
Health Quiz (total score on quiz, lower is better)	11	8	3

CHAPTER 10

Day 2 of The UltraSimple Diet

*"I lost 12 pounds, 2 inches off my waist,
1½ inches on my hips"*

*Having had a heart attack 10 years ago, high cholesterol,
triglycerides, and blood pressure and being overweight, I decided to give the program a try. Looking back now I am so
happy I did . . . I lost 12 pounds, 2 inches off my waist, 1½
inches off my hips. Before I went on The Ultra Simple Diet I
was tired and feeling old and cranky. The day couldn't end fast
enough. The amount of energy I have after 7 days is remarkable. I plan on making this my lifestyle, and if you knew me
seven days ago this was not my style.*

*P.S.: I just came back from my doctor (I go every month)
and he said my blood pressure was perfect and not to see him
for 4 months. Now that's progress.*

**Phil Solmonson
Melrose, MA**

Read Phil's whole story at the end of this chapter.

For more success stories, go to www.ultrasimplediet.com/success.

Today you might feel a little clearer, less puffy, though you still
may struggle a bit with fatigue and withdrawal symptoms. You
will be working through the hardest day. Hang in there. Get
enough rest. Eat frequently enough so you are not hungry. Be
kind to yourself.

Checklist for Day 2

If you don't want to write in your book, I have reprinted this checklist in the downloadable *UltraSimple Companion Guide* at www.ultrasimplediet.com/guide.

Action Items for Day 2 on the Program

☐ Wake up 90–120 minutes before you need to leave the house.

Upon Waking

☐ 2 tbsp. organic, extra-virgin olive oil mixed with the juice of ½ of an organic lemon—drink down to help flush the toxins from your bile and liver into your gut to be excreted

☐ 1 tsp. buffered ascorbic acid (vitamin C) powder in 8 ounces of water or 2–3 1000-mg capsules of buffered ascorbic acid (vitamin C)

Morning Ritual

☐ 20–60 minutes yoga

☐ **20 minutes journaling (You can do this by printing the journal in the downloadable guide at www.ultra simplediet.com/guide or in the online version of the community at www.ultrasimplediet.com/join.)**

Breakfast (7–9 a.m.)

☐ **Lemon juice (from ½ lemon) and hot water**

☐ **1 cup of green tea, steeped in hot water for 5 minutes (You may also have the green tea later in the day. Limit your intake to 2 cups a day.)**

☐ 2 capsules of probiotics before eating

☐ 2 capsules of liver supportive herbs and nutrients before eating

☐ **UltraShake**

☐ **If no bowel movement by 10 a.m., take herbal laxative (2–3 capsules). If no bowel movement in 6 hours, follow the steps for overcoming constipation in chapter 5.**

Morning Snack (10–11 a.m.)

☐ **1 cup UltraBroth**

☐ **Another UltraShake without flaxseeds or combination flax and borage oil (if you are hungry)**

Lunch (12–1 p.m.)

☐ 2 capsules or tablets of magnesium citrate with the meal (average capsule or tablet is 100–150 mg)

☐ **2 cups or more of steamed or lightly sautéed veggies (You should eat enough to feel gently satisfied.)**

☐ ½ cup cooked brown rice

☐ **½ cup fruit or berries for dessert (Either here or at dinner, not both, and only 1–2 times during the 7 day program.)**

☐ **UltraShake (optional)**

Afternoon Snack (2–3 p.m.)

☐ **1 cup UltraBroth**

☐ **UltraShake (if you are hungry)**

☐ Afternoon rest if possible for 30 minutes, or leisurely walk

Before Dinner

☐ 30-minute walk or aerobic exercise

☐ Sauna or steam at least 3 times a week if possible

☐ 20 minutes yoga

Dinner (5–7 p.m.)

- [ ] 2 capsules of probiotics before eating
- [ ] 2 capsules of liver detox supportive herbs and nutrients before eating
- [ ] **2 cups or more of steamed or lightly sautéed veggies (You should eat enough to feel gently satisfied.)**
- [ ] **½ cup of brown rice**
- [ ] **4–6 ounces of fish or chicken breast or 1 cup of legumes or tofu**
- [ ] **1 cup UltraBroth**

Bedtime or Evening Ritual

- [ ] 20 minutes restorative yoga
- [ ] **20 minutes journaling (if desired)**
- [ ] 2–3 capsules of herbal laxative (if no bowel movement that day)
- [ ] 2 capsules of magnesium citrate
- [ ] **20-minute UltraBath**
- [ ] **Interact with others, share tips, recipes and other advice in the UltraSimple community at www.ultra simplediet.com/join.**

* You can eat the lunch menu at dinner or the dinner menu at lunch, whatever is most convenient for you. Remember, if you prepare your food the night before, you can take it with you to work and just heat it up.

Journaling Exercises for Day 2

I've included a special section in the downloadable guide at www.ultrasimplediet.com/guide where you can keep track of your daily journaling activity. Print out the guide so you have an easy place to record your thoughts. Or, you can record them online by going to the special community at www.ultra simplediet.com/join.

In the Morning

Do this journaling exercise in the morning on the **second day** of the program:

- ⟡ What can I do today to truly take care of my body?
- ⟡ What can I do today to truly take care of my spirit?
- ⟡ What toxic food/idea/behavior can I do without today?

In the Evening

Do this exercise in the evening on the **second day** of the program.

- ⟡ What worked for me today?
- ⟡ What can I improve on tomorrow?
- ⟡ What symptoms improved today?
- ⟡ What did I notice about how I am feeling?
- ⟡ What did I learn today on the program that I can carry with me into the rest of my life?

UltraSimple Tip of the Day

Detox Tip: **Go Organic!**

Eat organic food and animal products to avoid petrochemical pesticides, herbicides, fumigants, hormones, and antibiotics.

Search out local markets for organic produce and animal produce, and whenever possible use certified organic fruits and vegetables. See www.ewg.org for more information on the most important organic products to eat.

For more tips on boosting your metabolism with the latest science, download *The UltraSimple Companion Guide* at www.ultrasimplediet.com/guide.

An UltraSimple Case Study

At the beginning I wondered if this program was for me. I'm a 58-year-old man who's used to eating meat, bread, and potatoes. Having had a heart attack 10 years ago, high cholesterol, triglycerides, and blood pressure, and being overweight, I decided to give it a try.

Looking back now I'm so happy I did. In just 7 days I lost 12 pounds, 2 inches off my waist, and 1½ inches off my hips.

My sinus problems cleared up, the swelling I used to have in both feet every night was gone, and my arthritis and joint pain seemed to have diminished. It wasn't gone entirely, but there was a vast improvement.

My alertness during the day improved, and my eyes seemed to be wide open. Before the program I was tired and feeling old, and cranky. It was like my day couldn't end fast enough. I would try to get everything done in the morning, so after lunch I could call it a day.

Now I wake up, and I'm ready to tackle the day. I do as much in the afternoon as in the morning. The amount of energy I have is remarkable.

I plan on making this my lifestyle and if you knew me seven days ago this was not my style.

P.S.: I just came back from my doctor (I go every month) and he said my blood pressure was perfect and not to see him for 4 months. Now that's progress.

Phil Solmonson
Melrose, MA

Here are Phil's measurements before and after the program.

Measurements	Before	After	Improvement
Weight (in pounds)	325	313	12
Waist (in inches)	59	56.75	2.25
Hips (in inches)	56.5	55.5	1
Health Quiz (total score on quiz, lower is better)	84	14	70

CHAPTER 11

Day 3 of The UltraSimple Diet

"I've lost 12 pounds and 4.5 percent body fat . . ."

After having my first child, I gained 40 pounds. After starting the UM diet in June, I lost a couple of pounds and ultimately began to feel better. But after blood tests in August, my cholesterol and C-reactive protein had changed little. My doctor gave me until early December to try to lower it some more before prescribing medication. I joined a Boot Camp–style workout and The UltraSimple Diet came along at a great time, right before my next blood test to see if I had improved any. I have lost 12 pounds and 4.5 percent body fat since exercising and dieting properly and my C-reactive protein count has dropped dramatically . . .

Victoria Stanbach
San Mateo, CA

Read Victoria's whole story at the end of this chapter.

For more success stories, go to www.ultrasimplediet.com/success.

Today you should start to emerge from the allergic and toxic fog you have been feeling for years, and should continue to lose weight. You should start to feel more energy and alertness. You might sleep better, and symptoms like pain, congestion and digestive distress should start to fade. You are in the home stretch. It just gets easier and better from here.

Checklist for Day 3

If you don't want to write in your book, I have reprinted this checklist in the downloadable *UltraSimple Companion Guide* at www.ultrasimplediet.com/guide.

Action Items for Day 3 on the Program

- [ ] Wake up 90–120 minutes before you need to leave the house.

Upon Waking

- [ ] 2 tbsp. organic, extra-virgin olive oil mixed with the juice of ½ of an organic lemon—drink down to help flush the toxins from your bile and liver into your gut to be excreted

- [ ] 1 tsp. buffered ascorbic acid (vitamin C) powder in 8 ounces of water or 2–3 1000-mg capsules of buffered ascorbic acid (vitamin C)

Morning Ritual

- [ ] 20–60 minutes yoga

- [ ] **20 minutes journaling (You can do this by printing the journal in the downloadable guide at www.ultra simplediet.com/guide or in the online version of the community at www.ultrasimplediet.com/join.)**

Breakfast (7–9 a.m.)

- [ ] **Lemon juice (from ½ lemon) and hot water**

- [ ] **1 cup of green tea, steeped in hot water for 5 minutes (You may also have the green tea later in the day. Limit your intake to 2 cups a day.)**

- [ ] 2 capsules of probiotics before eating

- [ ] 2 capsules of liver supportive herbs and nutrients before eating

- [ ] **UltraShake**

- [ ] **If no bowel movement by 10 a.m., take herbal laxative (2–3 capsules). If no bowel movement in 6 hours,**

follow the steps for overcoming constipation in
chapter 5.

Morning Snack (10–11 a.m.)

☐ **1 cup UltraBroth**

☐ **Another UltraShake without flaxseeds or combination
flax and borage oil (if you are hungry)**

Lunch (12–1 p.m.)

☐ 2 capsules or tablets of magnesium citrate with the meal
(average capsule or tablet is 100–150 mg)

☐ **2 cups or more of steamed or lightly sautéed veggies
(You should eat enough to feel gently satisfied.)**

☐ **½ cup cooked brown rice**

☐ ½ cup fruit or berries for dessert (Either here or at
dinner, not both, and only 1–2 times during the 7-day
program.)

☐ **UltraShake (optional)**

Afternoon Snack (2–3 p.m.)

☐ **1 cup UltraBroth**

☐ **UltraShake (if you are hungry)**

☐ Afternoon rest if possible for 30 minutes, or leisurely walk

Before Dinner

☐ 30-minute walk or aerobic exercise

☐ Sauna or steam at least 3 times a week if possible

☐ 20 minutes yoga

Dinner (5–7 p.m.)

☐ 2 capsules of probiotics before eating

☐ 2 capsules of liver detox supportive herbs and nutrients
before eating

- [ ] **2 cups or more of steamed or lightly sautéed veggies (You should eat enough to feel gently satisfied.)**
- [ ] **½ cup of brown rice**
- [ ] **4–6 ounces of fish or chicken breast or 1 cup of legumes or tofu**
- [ ] **1 cup UltraBroth**

Bedtime or Evening Ritual

- [ ] 20 minutes restorative yoga
- [ ] **20 minutes journaling (if desired)**
- [ ] 2–3 capsules of herbal laxative (if no bowel movement that day)
- [ ] 2 capsules of magnesium citrate
- [ ] **20-minute UltraBath**
- [ ] **Interact with others, share tips, recipes and other advice in the UltraSimple community at www.ultra simplediet.com/join.**

* You can eat the lunch menu at dinner or the dinner menu at lunch, whatever is most convenient for you. Remember, if you prepare your food the night before, you can take it with you to work and just heat it up.

Journaling Exercises for Day 3

I've included a special section in the downloadable guide at www.ultrasimplediet.com/guide where you can keep track of your daily journaling activity. Print out the guide so you have an easy place to record your thoughts. Or, you can record them online by going to the special community at www.ultra simplediet.com/join.

In the Morning

Do this journaling exercise in the morning on the **third day** of the program:

✧ What can I do today to truly take care of my body?
✧ What can I do today to truly take care of my spirit?
✧ What toxic food/idea/behavior can I do without today?

In the Evening

Do this exercise in the evening on the **third day** of the program:

✧ What worked for me today?
✧ What can I improve on tomorrow?
✧ What symptoms improved today?
✧ What did I notice about how I am feeling?
✧ What did I learn today on the program that I can carry with me into the rest of my life?

UltraSimple Tip of the Day

Inflammation Tip: **The Power of Touch**

Historically touch has always been thought to have healing powers. Intuitively we recognize the power of touch to heal. We often stroke a child's forehead when he or she is sick, or rub a part of our body when it is sore. Now there is science to back up this idea.

The power of touch can have almost magical anti-inflammatory properties. If you want to reduce the inflammation in your body, you can try touch therapy.

One wonderful way to do this is by having a massage. If you can't afford a professional massage during your 7-day program, trade massages with a friend or your spouse. It may help reduce you inflammation and is also wonderfully relaxing.

For more tips on boosting your metabolism with the latest science, download *The UltraSimple Companion Guide* at www.ultrasimplediet.com/guide.

An UltraSimple Case Study

I started the program, because the checkup I had a year before scared me. My doctor told me I had high cholesterol and my C-reactive protein (the best indicator for how inflamed you are) was off the charts. A healthy score is below 1. I scored 10.5.

She also detected a heart murmur which was . . . interesting. I had been feeling heart palpitations and chest pain, but I couldn't figure out if I was making it all up.

My doctor gave me until December to get my health in order or she was going to prescribe medication, and I was not thrilled about the idea of being on cholesterol meds.

I knew I was overweight, and I knew that was contributing to my health problems. I put on about 40 pounds after my son was born, and I had a really hard time losing it. Nothing I did seemed to make any difference.

Then I found the UltraMetabolism diet in June. I lost a couple of pounds, and ultimately began to feel better.

I joined a Boot Camp–style workout, and The UltraSimple Diet came along at a great time—right before my next blood test.

Since following this program and exercising I have lost 12 pounds, and 4.5 percent of my body fat. That didn't all happen in one week, but the 7-day program jumpstarted the change.

What's more, my C-reactive protein measurement dropped to 7.1 over the course of one week on the program. That's not where it needs to be, but it's a huge improvement for one week.

This program has given me the information I need to get my health back on track.

Victoria Stanbach
San Mateo, CA

Here are Victoria's measurements before and after the program.

Measurements	Before	After	Improvement
Weight (in pounds)	217	213	4
Waist (in inches)	43.25	42	1.25
Hips (in inches)	44.25	44	.25
Health Quiz (total score on quiz, lower is better)	55	21	34

CHAPTER 12

Day 4 of The UltraSimple Diet

*". . . what truly amazes me is how much my health
has improved. I stopped taking almost all
of the medicine I was on."*

*I lost 7 pounds, I look better, and that feels great. But what
truly amazes me is how much my health has improved. I stopped
taking almost all of the medicine I was on. I've been trying to
lose weight for so long, and nothing was working. Today I feel
like I have been reborn. The program is that powerful.*

**Billie Mann
Kansas City, MO**

Read Billie's whole story at the end of this chapter.

For more success stories, go to www.ultrasimplediet.com/success.

You are more than halfway there. Now the benefits should start
to increase. The cravings should be gone. Your energy should
increase. Your brain fog and postnasal drip should clear up.
You should pay attention to your sensations, feelings, and the
taste of food. You will still need rest and care. So don't spend
all your new energy, save it.

Checklist for Day 4

If you don't want to write in your book, I have reprinted this
checklist in the downloadable *UltraSimple Companion Guide*
at www.ultrasimplediet.com/guide.

Action Items for Day 4 on the Program

☐ Wake up 90–120 minutes before you need to leave the house.

Upon Waking

☐ 2 tbsp. organic extra-virgin olive oil mixed with the juice of ½ of an organic lemon—drink down to help flush the toxins from your bile and liver into your gut to be excreted

☐ 1 tsp. buffered ascorbic acid (vitamin C) powder in 8 ounces of water or 2–3 1000-mg capsules of buffered ascorbic acid (vitamin C)

Morning Ritual

☐ 20–60 minutes yoga

☐ **20 minutes journaling (You can do this by printing the journal in the downloadable guide at www.ultra simplediet.com/guide or in the online version of the community at www.ultrasimplediet.com/join.)**

Breakfast (7–9 a.m.)

☐ **Lemon juice (from ½ lemon) and hot water**

☐ **1 cup of green tea, steeped in hot water for 5 minutes (You may also have the green tea later in the day. Limit your intake to 2 cups a day.)**

☐ 2 capsules of probiotics before eating

☐ 2 capsules of liver supportive herbs and nutrients before eating

☐ **UltraShake**

☐ **If no bowel movement by 10 a.m., take herbal laxative (2–3 capsules). If no bowel movement in 6 hours, follow the steps for overcoming constipation in chapter 5.**

Morning Snack (10–11 a.m.)

- [ ] **1 cup UltraBroth**
- [ ] **Another UltraShake without flaxseeds or combination flax and borage oil (if you are hungry)**

Lunch (12–1 p.m.)

- [ ] 2 capsules or tablets of magnesium citrate with the meal (average capsule or tablet is 100–150 mg)
- [ ] **2 cups or more of steamed or lightly sautéed veggies (You should eat enough to feel gently satisfied.)**
- [ ] **½ cup cooked brown rice**
- [ ] **½ cup fruit or berries for dessert (Either here or at dinner, not both, and only 1–2 times during the 7-day program.)**
- [ ] **UltraShake (optional)**

Afternoon Snack (2–3 p.m.)

- [ ] **1 cup UltraBroth**
- [ ] **UltraShake (if you are hungry)**
- [ ] Afternoon rest if possible for 30 minutes, or leisurely walk

Before Dinner

- [ ] 30-minute walk or aerobic exercise
- [ ] Sauna or steam at least 3 times a week if possible
- [ ] 20 minutes yoga

Dinner (5–7 p.m.)

- [ ] 2 capsules of probiotics before eating
- [ ] 2 capsules of liver detox supportive herbs and nutrients before eating
- [ ] **2 cups or more of steamed or lightly sautéed veggies (You should eat enough to feel gently satisfied.)**

☐   ½ cup of brown rice

☐   **4–6 ounces of fish or chicken breast or 1 cup of legumes or tofu**

☐   **1 cup UltraBroth**

Bedtime or Evening Ritual

☐   20 minutes restorative yoga

☐   **20 minutes journaling (if desired)**

☐   2–3 capsules of herbal laxative (if no bowel movement that day)

☐   2 capsules of magnesium citrate

☐   **20-minute UltraBath**

☐   **Interact with others, share tips, recipes and other advice in the UltraSimple community at www.ultra simplediet.com/join.**

* You can eat the lunch menu at dinner or the dinner menu at lunch, whatever is most convenient for you. Remember, if you prepare your food the night before, you can take it with you to work and just heat it up.

Journaling Exercises for Day 4

I've included a special section in the downloadable guide at www.ultrasimplediet.com/guide where you can keep track of your daily journaling activity. Print out the guide so you have an easy place to record your thoughts. Or, you can record them online by going to the special community at www.ultra simplediet.com/join.

In the Morning

Do this journaling exercise in the morning on the **fourth day** of the program:

- ✧ What can I do today to truly take care of my body?
- ✧ What can I do today to truly take care of my spirit?
- ✧ What toxic food/idea/behavior can I do without today?

In the Evening

Do this exercise in the evening on the **fourth day** of the program.

- ✧ What worked for me today?
- ✧ What can I improve on tomorrow?
- ✧ What symptoms improved today?
- ✧ What did I notice about how I am feeling?
- ✧ What did I learn today on the program that I can carry with me into the rest of my life?

UltraSimple Tip of the Day

Sleep Tip: **Create a Sleep Ritual**

Good sleep is not something that just happens (unless you are a baby or a teenager). There are clearly defined things that interfere with or support healthy sleep. So don't expect to just hop into bed, shut your eyes, and go out like a light if you aren't used to doing that or haven't set the stage for good sleep.

Try taking a little "holiday" 2 hours before you go to bed. Create a ritual of special little things you do during this time to help set the stage for sleep. Turn off the TV and computer, listen to soothing music, do a little yoga or stretching, or take an UltraBath. This helps your system prepare physically and psychologically for sleep, and can guide your body into a deep, healing sleep.

For more tips on boosting your metabolism with the latest science, download *The UltraSimple Companion Guide* at www.ultrasimplediet.com/guide.

An UltraSimple Case Study

I'm diabetic, overweight, suffer from GERD, chronic fatigue syndrome, and Epstein-Barr virus, and I was depressed. I've been an energetic woman my whole life. I raised four children and work a full-time job. But now I was completely exhausted all the time. I was taking handfuls of pills morning and night, but they didn't improve my condition any. And despite regular diet and exercise I hadn't lost a single pound for over 3 years.

I felt like I was a burden to my husband and children. They worried about me all the time, and I was terrified they would eventually be forced to put me in a nursing home. It was getting that bad.

I needed something to kick-start my body into reversing the trend it was on. This program has done that.

I lost 7 pounds, I look better, and that feels great. But what truly amazes me is how much my health has improved. I stopped taking almost all of the medicine I was on. And now, even though the program is over, I only need to take 3 or 4 pills a day.

I've been trying to lose weight for so long, and nothing was working. Today I feel like I have been reborn. The program is that powerful.

Billie Mann
Kansas City, MO

Here are Billie's measurements before and after the program.

Measurements	Before	After	Improvement
Weight (in pounds)	198	191	7
Waist (in inches)	32.5	30	2.5
Hips (in inches)	43	40.5	2.5
Health Quiz (total score on quiz, lower is better)	138	9	129

CHAPTER 13

Day 5 of The UltraSimple Diet

"I'm embarrassed to say this, but I'm a doctor and I didn't make the connection between what I ate, how I treated my body, and my health until it was almost too late."

On the UltraSimple program I lost 4 pounds, which made me feel great. My back pain almost went away completely, and I feel more energetic and healthier than I have in years. I'm embarrassed to say this, but I'm a doctor and I didn't make the connection between what I ate, how I treated my body, and my health until it was almost too late.

Elizabeth Neel
Raleigh, NC

Read Elizabeth's whole story at the end of this chapter.

For more success stories, go to www.ultrasimplediet.com/success.

Today begin to check in more closely with your body and your mind. Have you noticed you feel more even tempered, less moody, more positive? Your emotions are directly connected to your diet and your stress level. Notice the difference just 5 days makes.

Checklist for Day 5

If you don't want to write in your book, I have reprinted this checklist in the downloadable *UltraSimple Companion Guide* at www.ultrasimplediet.com/guide.

Action Items for Day 5 on the Program

☐ Wake up 90–120 minutes before you need to leave the house.

Upon Waking

☐ 2 tbsp. organic extra-virgin olive oil mixed with the juice of ½ of an organic lemon—drink down to help flush the toxins from your bile and liver into your gut to be excreted

☐ 1 tsp. buffered ascorbic acid (vitamin C) powder in 8 ounces of water or 2–3 1000-mg capsules of buffered ascorbic acid (vitamin C)

Morning Ritual

☐ 20–60 minutes yoga

☐ **20 minutes journaling (You can do this by printing the journal in the downloadable guide at www.ultra simplediet.com/guide or in the online version of the community at www.ultrasimplediet.com/join.)**

Breakfast (7-9 a.m.)

☐ **Lemon juice (from ½ lemon) and hot water**

☐ **1 cup of green tea, steeped in hot water for 5 minutes (You may also have the green tea later in the day. Limit your intake to 2 cups a day.)**

☐ 2 capsules of probiotics before eating

☐ 2 capsules of liver supportive herbs and nutrients before eating

☐ **UltraShake**

☐ **If no bowel movement by 10 a.m., take herbal laxative (2–3 capsules). If no bowel movement in 6 hours, follow the steps for overcoming constipation in chapter 5.**

Morning Snack (10–11 a.m.)

- [ ] **1 cup UltraBroth**
- [ ] **Another UltraShake without flaxseeds or combination flax and borage oil (if you are hungry)**

Lunch (12–1 p.m.)

- [ ] 2 capsules or tablets of magnesium citrate with the meal (average capsule or tablet is 100–150 mg)
- [ ] **2 cups or more of steamed or lightly sautéed veggies (You should eat enough to feel gently satisfied.)**
- [ ] ½ cup cooked brown rice
- [ ] ½ cup fruit or berries for dessert (Either here or at dinner, not both, and only 1–2 times during the 7-day program.)
- [ ] **UltraShake (optional)**

Afternoon Snack (2–3 p.m.)

- [ ] **1 cup UltraBroth**
- [ ] **UltraShake (if you are hungry)**
- [ ] Afternoon rest if possible for 30 minutes, or leisurely walk

Before Dinner

- [ ] 30-minute walk or aerobic exercise
- [ ] Sauna or steam at least 3 times a week if possible
- [ ] 20 minutes yoga

Dinner (5–7 p.m.)

- [ ] 2 capsules of probiotics before eating
- [ ] 2 capsules of liver detox supportive herbs and nutrients before eating
- [ ] **2 cups or more of steamed or lightly sautéed veggies (You should eat enough to feel gently satisfied.)**
- [ ] **½ cup of brown rice**

☐ **4–6 ounces of fish or chicken breast or 1 cup of legumes or tofu**

☐ **1 cup UltraBroth**

Bedtime or Evening Ritual

☐ 20 minutes restorative yoga

☐ **20 minutes journaling (if desired)**

☐ 2–3 capsules of herbal laxative (if no bowel movement that day)

☐ 2 capsules of magnesium citrate

☐ **20-minute UltraBath**

☐ **Interact with others, share tips, recipes and other advice in the UltraSimple community at www.ultra simplediet.com/join.**

* You can eat the lunch menu at dinner or the dinner menu at lunch, whatever is most convenient for you. Remember, if you prepare your food the night before, you can take it with you to work and just heat it up.

Journaling Exercises for Day 5

I've included a special section in the downloadable guide at www.ultrasimplediet.com/guide where you can keep track of your daily journaling activity. Print out the guide so you have an easy place to record your thoughts. Or, you can record them online by going to the special community at www.ultra simplediet.com/join.

In the Morning

Do this journaling exercise in the morning on the **fifth day** of the program:

✧ What can I do today to truly take care of my body?

✧ What can I do today to truly take care of my spirit?

✧ What toxic food/idea/behavior can I do without today?

In the Evening

Do this exercise in the evening on the **fifth day** of the program.

- ✧ What worked for me today?
- ✧ What can I improve on tomorrow?
- ✧ What symptoms improved today?
- ✧ What did I notice about how I am feeling?
- ✧ What did I learn today on the program that I can carry with me into the rest of my life?

UltraSimple Tip of the Day

Supplement Tip: **Magnesium**

Magnesium is the relaxation mineral. Our processed diet contains almost no magnesium. If you have a twitch, a spasm, a cramp, or an irritable something, the chances are you are very low on magnesium.

You can't afford to miss out on your magnesium. It is critical for more than 300 chemical processes in your body.

For long-term health you should consider taking a magnesium supplement permanently.

For more tips on boosting your metabolism with the latest science (and for more information in this specific supplement), download *The UltraSimple Companion Guide* at www.ultrasimplediet.com/guide.

An UltraSimple Case Study

About a year ago I hit bottom. I had a miscarriage, and complications led me into surgery. Then I injured my back so badly that pain radiated through my hips, down my leg, and my foot went numb. I had to go on steroids, and a host of other medications, and that made the pounds start piling on.

It shook me to the core. I thought, "I'm 36, and I'm starting to circle the drain. All those years of neglect are coming back to haunt me. I don't exercise or eat well. I'm constantly stressed out. And I take medication all the time, but I don't get any better. I'm pitiful. Something has to change."

Frankly, it's a bit ironic. I'm embarrassed to say this, but I'm a doctor and I didn't make the connection between what I ate, how I treated my body, and my health until it was almost too late.

On the UltraSimple program I lost 4 pounds, which was amazing. My back pain almost went away completely, and I feel more energetic and healthier than I have in years.

Having been a "traditionally" trained doctor, I was always skeptical of "alternative" approaches. Dr. Hyman has given me a new respect for the holistic approach, and a deeper understanding of nutrition and the body.

Elizabeth Neel
Raleigh, NC

Here are Elizabeth's measurements before and after the program.

Measurements	Before	After	Improvement
Weight (in pounds)	156.6	152	4.6
Waist (in inches)	34	33.75	.25
Hips (in inches)	39.5	38.5	1
Health Quiz (total score on quiz, lower is better)	64	44	20

CHAPTER 14

Day 6 of The UltraSimple Diet

*"I CANNOT believe it! I lost 16 pounds and
3 inches off my waist in one week!"*

*I CANNOT believe it! I lost 16 pounds and 3 inches off my
waist in one week! I had so much toxic fluid I would never have
known about if it wasn't for this book. Thank you, Dr. Hyman.
This one week gave me the motivation to continue, and your
information gave me the tools.*

**Diane Rupinski
Woodstock, CT**

Read Diane's whole story at the end of this chapter.

For more success stories, go to www.ultrasimplediet.com/success.

You are almost through the program. The benefits should
be building. You might be tempted to cheat because you feel so
good, or to overdo it with activities because you haven't had so
much energy in years, but stay with it. Your body and your metabolism are just beginning to reset and the best is yet to come.

Checklist for Day 6

If you don't want to write in your book, I have reprinted this
checklist in the downloadable *UltraSimple Companion Guide*
at www.ultrasimplediet.com/guide.

Action Items for Day 6 on the Program

☐ Wake up 90–120 minutes before you need to leave the house.

Upon Waking

☐ 2 tbsp. organic, extra-virgin olive oil mixed with the juice of ½ of an organic lemon—drink down to help flush the toxins from your bile and liver into your gut to be excreted

☐ 1 tsp. buffered ascorbic acid (vitamin C) powder in 8 ounces of water or 2–3 1000-mg capsules of buffered ascorbic acid (vitamin C)

Morning Ritual

☐ 20–60 minutes yoga

☐ **20 minutes journaling (You can do this by printing the journal in the downloadable guide at www.ultra simplediet.com/guide or in the online version of the community at www.ultrasimplediet.com/join.)**

Breakfast (7–9 a.m.)

☐ **Lemon juice (from ½ lemon) and hot water**

☐ **1 cup of green tea, steeped in hot water for 5 minutes (You may also have the green tea later in the day. Limit your intake to 2 cups a day.)**

☐ 2 capsules of probiotics before eating

☐ 2 capsules of liver supportive herbs and nutrients before eating

☐ **UltraShake**

☐ **If no bowel movement by 10 a.m., take herbal laxative (2–3 capsules). If no bowel movement in 6 hours, follow the steps for overcoming constipation in chapter 5.**

Morning Snack (10–11 a.m.)

- [ ] **1 cup UltraBroth**
- [ ] **Another UltraShake without flaxseeds or combination flax and borage oil (if you are hungry)**

Lunch (12–1 p.m.)

- [ ] **2 capsules or tablets of magnesium citrate with the meal (average capsule or tablet is 100–150 mg)**
- [ ] **2 cups or more of steamed or lightly sautéed veggies (You should eat enough to feel gently satisfied.)**
- [ ] **½ cup cooked brown rice**
- [ ] **½ cup fruit or berries for dessert (Either here or at dinner, not both, and only 1–2 times during the 7-day program.)**
- [ ] **UltraShake (optional)**

Afternoon Snack (2–3 p.m.)

- [ ] **1 cup UltraBroth**
- [ ] **UltraShake (if you are hungry)**
- [ ] Afternoon rest if possible for 30 minutes, or leisurely walk

Before Dinner

- [ ] 30-minute walk or aerobic exercise
- [ ] Sauna or steam at least 3 times a week if possible
- [ ] 20 minutes yoga

Dinner (5–7 p.m.)

- [ ] 2 capsules of probiotics before eating
- [ ] 2 capsules of liver detox supportive herbs and nutrients before eating
- [ ] **2 cups or more of steamed or lightly sautéed veggies (You should eat enough to feel gently satisfied.)**

- ☐ ½ cup of brown rice
- ☐ **4–6 ounces of fish or chicken breast or 1 cup of legumes or tofu**
- ☐ **1 cup UltraBroth**

Bedtime or Evening Ritual

- ☐ 20 minutes restorative yoga
- ☐ **20 minutes journaling (if desired)**
- ☐ 2–3 capsules of herbal laxative (if no bowel movement that day)
- ☐ 2 capsules of magnesium citrate
- ☐ **20-minute UltraBath**
- ☐ **Interact with others, share tips, recipes and other advice in the UltraSimple community at www.ultra simplediet.com/join.**

* You can eat the lunch menu at dinner or the dinner menu at lunch, whatever is most convenient for you. Remember, if you prepare your food the night before, you can take it with you to work and just heat it up.

Journaling Exercises for Day 6

I've included a special section in the downloadable guide at www.ultrasimplediet.com/guide where you can keep track of your daily journaling activity. Print out the guide so you have an easy place to record your thoughts. Or, you can record them online by going to the special community at www.ultra simplediet.com/join.

In the Morning

Do this journaling exercise in the morning on the **sixth day** of the program:

- ✧ What can I do today to truly take care of my body?
- ✧ What can I do today to truly take care of my spirit?

✧ What toxic food / idea / behavior can I do without today?

In the Evening

Do this exercises in the evening on the **sixth day** of the program.

✧ What worked for me today?
✧ What can I improve on tomorrow?
✧ What symptoms improved today?
✧ What did I notice about how I am feeling?
✧ What did I learn today on the program that I can carry with me into the rest of my life?

UltraSimple Tip of the Day

Exercise Tip: **Improving Cardio**

I recommend you begin a regular regimen of cardiovascular exercise. Here are some tips on how to get started:

✦ Try walking to start—even just 5 minutes a day is good to begin with.
✦ Experiment with different forms of exercise: walking, swimming, aerobics, jogging, Rollerblading, jumping rope, rowing, cycling, spinning, exercise machines, cross-country skiing, skating, kick boxing, dancing, rebounding on a mini trampoline, hiking a mountain, or anything else that grabs you
✦ Try to exercise in the fresh air if possible.
✦ Be sure to increase your level of exertion as your fitness level improves. If you stay at that same speed and

incline on the treadmill for years without increasing
your effort, your benefits go downhill.

✦ Build up slowly to 30 minutes a day of vigorous
cardiovascular exercise.

For more tips on boosting your metabolism with the latest
science, download *The UltraSimple Companion Guide* at
www.ultrasimplediet.com/guide.

An UltraSimple Case Study

*When I learned about the program I was overweight, suffered
from terrible sinus problems, and had recurring GI issues.
I didn't sleep well, I woke up groggy, my body ached, my
face was bloated, and my eyes were constantly swollen. I
needed some serious motivation to get my health back on track
again.*

*When I got on the scale after 7 days on the program I
thought, "I CANNOT believe it!"*

I lost 16 pounds and 3 inches off my waist in one week!

*The overall improvement in my health was pretty astound-
ing as well. My sinus problems and GI problems disappeared.
The bloating in my face was gone, and my eyes are no longer
swollen. I sleep better, wake up alert, and my energy has sky-
rocketed. On day 6 of the program I found myself easily doing
chores in my garden I would have had a very hard time accom-
plishing before.*

*The improvement in my overall sense of health and well-
being is tremendous. And I have been able to keep the weight
off months after the 7 days ended.*

*This one week gave me the motivation to want to continue.
The information I learned gave me the tools to do it.*

**Diane Rupinski
Raleigh, NC**

Here are Diane's measurements before and after the program.

Measurements	Before	After	Improvement
Weight (in pounds)	231	215	16
Waist (in inches)	43	40	3
Hips (in inches)	53	50	3
Health Quiz (total score on quiz, lower is better)	113	82	31

CHAPTER 15

Day 7 of The UltraSimple Diet

> *"I cannot believe how strong I feel,*
> *full of energy and vitality."*

Eating all the varieties of foods including the UltraBroth and the UltraShake gave me more energy than I have ever had before. It was like my body clock turned back time. I feel younger and healthier. Within one week on the program I lost 5 pounds. I cannot believe how strong I feel, full of energy and vitality. This has been a very exciting and healing experience.

Esther Suen
Daly City, CA

Read Esther's whole story at the end of this chapter.

For more success stories, go to www.ultrasimplediet.com/success.

Stop. Close your eyes. Notice and slowly scan every part of your body from your head to your toes. How different do you feel from a week ago? How is your energy? How is your mood? Are your clothes loose?

Today you will finish the program. You should be a different person than when you started. Now you have the opportunity to carry this into the rest of your life. Follow the recommendations about how to transition out of the program if you want to continue to feel good and get the maximum benefit from all the work you have done.

Checklist for Day 7

If you don't want to write in your book, I have reprinted this checklist in the downloadable *UltraSimple Companion Guide* at www.ultrasimplediet.com/guide.

Action Items for Day 7 on the Program

☐ Wake up 90–120 minutes before you need to leave the house.

Upon Waking

☐ 2 tbsp. organic, extra-virgin olive oil mixed with the juice of ½ of an organic lemon—drink down to help flush the toxins from your bile and liver into your gut to be excreted

☐ 1 tsp. buffered ascorbic acid (vitamin C) powder in 8 ounces of water or 2–3 1000-mg capsules of buffered ascorbic acid (vitamin C)

Morning Ritual

☐ 20–60 minutes yoga

☐ **20 minutes journaling (You can do this by printing the journal in the downloadable guide at www.ultrasimplediet.com/guide or in the online version of the community at www.ultrasimplediet.com/join.)**

Breakfast (7–9 a.m.)

☐ **Lemon juice (from ½ lemon) and hot water**

☐ **1 cup of green tea, steeped in hot water for 5 minutes (You may also have the green tea later in the day. Limit your intake to 2 cups a day.)**

☐ 2 capsules of probiotics before eating

☐ 2 capsules of liver supportive herbs and nutrients before eating

☐ **UltraShake**

☐ **If no bowel movement by 10 a.m., take herbal laxative (2–3 capsules). If no bowel movement in 6 hours, follow the steps for overcoming constipation in chapter 5.**

Morning Snack (10–11 a.m.)

☐ **1 cup UltraBroth**

☐ **Another UltraShake without flaxseeds or combination flax and borage oil (if you are hungry)**

Lunch (12–1 p.m.)

☐ 2 capsules or tablets of magnesium citrate with the meal (average capsule or tablet is 100–150 mg)

☐ **2 cups or more of steamed or lightly sautéed veggies (You should eat enough to feel gently satisfied.)**

☐ **½ cup cooked brown rice**

☐ **½ cup fruit or berries for dessert (Either here or at dinner, not both, and only 1–2 times during the 7-day program.)**

☐ **UltraShake (optional)**

Afternoon Snack (2–3 p.m.)

☐ **1 cup UltraBroth**

☐ **UltraShake (if you are hungry)**

☐ Afternoon rest if possible for 30 minutes, or leisurely walk

Before Dinner

☐ 30-minute walk or aerobic exercise

☐ Sauna or steam at least 3 times a week if possible

☐ 20 minutes yoga

Dinner (5–7 p.m.)

- [ ] 2 capsules of probiotics before eating
- [ ] 2 capsules of liver detox supportive herbs and nutrients before eating
- [ ] **2 cups or more of steamed or lightly sautéed veggies (You should eat enough to feel gently satisfied.)**
- [ ] **½ cup of brown rice**
- [ ] **4–6 ounces of fish or chicken breast or 1 cup of legumes or tofu**
- [ ] **1 cup UltraBroth**

Bedtime or Evening Ritual

- [ ] 20 minutes restorative yoga
- [ ] **20 minutes journaling (if desired)**
- [ ] 2–3 capsules of herbal laxative (if no bowel movement that day)
- [ ] 2 capsules of magnesium citrate
- [ ] **20-minute UltraBath**
- [ ] **Interact with others, share tips, recipes and other advice in the UltraSimple community at www.ultra simplediet.com/join.**

* You can eat the lunch menu at dinner or the dinner menu at lunch, whatever is most convenient for you. Remember, if you prepare your food the night before, you can take it with you to work and just heat it up.

Journaling Exercises for Day 7

I've included a special section in the downloadable guide at www.ultrasimplediet.com/guide where you can keep track of your daily journaling activity. Print out the guide so you have an easy place to record your thoughts. Or, you can record them online by going to the special community at www.ultra simplediet.com/join.

In the Morning

Do this journaling exercise in the morning on the **last day** of
the program:

- ◇ What can I do today to truly take care of my body?
- ◇ What can I do today to truly take care of my spirit?
- ◇ What toxic food / idea / behavior can I do without
  today?
- ◇ How do I feel today, physically?

In the Evening

Do this exercise in the evening on the **last day** of the program.

- ◇ What, if anything, do I notice about my body that is
  different than when this program started?
- ◇ If my body could speak, what story would it tell
  about this experience?
- ◇ How do I feel today, emotionally and spiritually?
- ◇ What, if anything, do I notice about my internal state
  that is different than when this program started?
- ◇ If my heart could speak, what story would it tell
  about this experience?
- ◇ What did I learn over the course of the program that
  I can carry with me into the rest of my life?

UltraSimple Tip of the Day

Stress Tip: **Breathe from Your Belly**

Restricted or shallow breathing prevents oxygen from
reaching all your tissues and can profoundly affect your en-

ergy. Learning to breathe properly is a quick trick to healing and relaxation. It is the easiest doorway to deep relaxation and can be done anywhere, anytime of the day, even in short little bursts.

Here's what to do:

Put your hand on your belly. Breathe out, squeezing the air out of your lungs with your stomach muscles. As you breathe in, relax your stomach muscles, and after you fill your lungs try to push your hand off your belly with your breath. Continue breathing in and out slowly through your nose. Each in and out breath should last to the count of three. Do this for 5 minutes a day, or whenever you feel stressed. It can save you in all sorts of situations. A full belly breath moves eight to ten times as much air as a chest breath!

For more tips on boosting your metabolism with the latest science, download *The UltraSimple Companion Guide* at www.ultrasimplediet.com/guide.

An UltraSimple Case Study

I had sweet cravings that would not stop. I love to make muffins and fruit pies for friends and family. Of course, I enjoyed them too. And when the box of donuts was passed around at work I couldn't help but eat a bit. I guess that's why I ended up 10 pounds overweight.

But the real reason I started the UltraSimple program was because I wanted to identify what in my diet was causing an itchy, flaky rash over my eyes. I was pretty sure it was related to food, but I wasn't exactly certain which foods were causing it.

In 7 days I lost 5 pounds, and my cravings for sweets completely dissolved. That was pretty unbelievable, because I used to eat sweets almost every day.

Eating all the varieties of foods including the UltraBroth and the UltraShake gave me more energy than I have ever had before. It was like my body clock turned back time. I feel younger and healthier.

I decided to reintroduce foods slowly after 7 days were over, so I could identify what was causing the rash over my eyes.

As a result I lost an additional 4 pounds (which brings me really close to my ideal weight!), and I've figured out that it's probably dairy, nuts, and MSG that cause the rash.

This has been a very healing experience for me. I feel more in control of what I eat, I can't believe how strong I feel, full of energy and vitality. I feel more in control of my body.

Esther Suen
Daly City, CA

Here are Esther's measurements before and after the program.

Measurements	Before	After	Improvement
Weight (in pounds)	137	132	5
Waist (in inches)	33	30	3
Hips (in inches)	41	39	2
Health Quiz (total score on quiz, lower is better)	26	5	21

Summary

✧ You have learned the day–by–day, step–by–step program for regaining your health in a very short time—7 days—and safely losing up to 10 pounds.

✧ Little things we can add to our life, from supplements to exercise to stress management tools to tips for detoxifying and reducing inflammation, can all enhance the quality of your health and your life.

What's Next

In the next chapter you will learn how to successfully transition out of the program and embark on a program of continued weight loss and lifelong health.

CHAPTER 16

How to Transition Out of The UltraSimple Diet

". . . this program showed me that there is hope for me."

When I started the UltraSimple program, I was really hoping to just lose some weight. I had previously tried a low-carb diet, and it took me 3 months to lose 6 pounds. My skin was a mess, and I really did not feel my best on this type of diet. Before I started the UltraSimple program, I took the health quiz and scored an 80. The program was very easy to follow and I feel planning and preparing the food ahead of time, as suggested, was the reason I was able to do the program so easily. During the program, I felt great, no bloating, no gas, no headaches or clogged sinuses (all of which I have on a regular basis). The best part for me was my skin clearing up. The added bonus besides feeling really good was a 5-pound weight loss. This is a real triumph for me. It normally takes me a very long time to lose any weight and I consequently give up. I have a lot of weight to lose, and this program showed me that there is hope for me. When I took the health quiz after one week I scored a 24, and I had lost 1½ inches around my waist and 1¾ inches around my hips . . .

Elise Schindler
Pittsburgh, PA

For more success stories, go to www.ultrasimplediet.com/success.

————————

In this chapter you will learn:

◇ How to successfully transition out of the program and embark on a program of continued weight loss and lifelong health

————————

The first thing to do as you complete your 7-day program is retake the "Toxicity and Inflammation Quiz." Complete the rest of the steps as outlined in chapter 2, including completing the rest of your vitals, taking your optional "after" picture, and shooting your optional "after" video where you tell the world and remind yourself about your success.

You can also either download *The UltraSimple Companion Guide* at www.ultrasimplediet.com/guide and complete your follow-up stats there or complete them online in the community at www.ultrasimplediet.com/join.

Compare your results with the ones you obtained before you began. You will soon see the magnitude of your newfound vitality and health. This should inspire you to continue on your path to lifelong, vital health—an UltraWellness lifestyle. But most importantly, you should FEEL better.

As you transition out of this week of healing, I encourage you to go slowly and savor the full benefits of the program.

The temptation will be to splurge or reward yourself for your hard work, but resist that temptation. Overloading your system with foods that you are allergic to, or with sugar, caffeine, and alcohol can often cause severe reactions.

Take it slowly, and choose what you really want carefully. Think about what was just a bad habit. Your body has wisdom that will awaken during your experience on the program. Listen to the wisdom of your body when creating your life after the program has ended. Go slowly and monitor your responses.

What to Do When the Program Is Over?

When your week-long program is over, you can (and should) continue many of the healthy habits you learned on the program so you can achieve UltraWellness, which is a lifestyle of optimal health. At this point you have two options. There actually IS a third option, one that gives you the best chance at making your health and weight improvement permanent and achieving UltraWellness, but I've saved that for the last chapter.

Option 1: Continue the Program

You may choose to keep doing the program until you achieve your ideal weight or desired health benefits.

Doing the program for an additional three weeks is ideal, but you may continue the program for a full 3 months if you choose. After 3 months you may be able to tolerate foods you are sensitive to as long as you only eat them occasionally—such as every 3–4 days.

In addition to the other dietary recommendations on this program, you should start the basic supplement plan I recommend that includes a multivitamin and mineral, calcium, magnesium, and vitamin D, and omega-3 fats if you have not already done so. I also recommend taking a probiotic regularly, but it is not absolutely necessary. Remember, these supplements are the foundation for long-term health.

You can also continue using the enhanced supplements for a total of 3 months to extend the benefits of that program if you choose to. This is not necessary, but the supplements can help support your efforts to further detoxify and reduce inflammation in your body.

After 3 months you should stop using these supplements. You will have done your body a great service. At that point much healing will have occurred and you may not need the enhanced supplements any longer.

You should only use the olive oil and lemon juice flush for one week—although you might want to make a habit of repeating the program one week every 3 months to give your system a healthy boost.

You may also choose to integrate pieces of the enhanced plan if you have been doing the basic plan up to this point.

For example, exercise and relaxation techniques may help you improve your results regardless of what program you have been practicing. If you have not already integrated these parts of the program into your daily routine, you may consider doing that now.

Option 2: End the Program, Reintegrate Foods, and Keep Your Healthy Lifestyle

If you are satisfied with the results you achieved on the 7-day program, you may choose to end the program now. However, there are a number of things to keep in mind. You don't want to simply go back to your old ways of eating and behaving. After all, you have suffered the consequences of that lifestyle for too long, and now you have the information you need to make healthy changes in your life.

If you do choose to end the program, there are a number of elements you may want to retain over the long term.

The basic supplement plan is one of them. As I have said throughout this book, using the basic supplement plan I outline is critical for long-term health and weight loss.

You can also continue enjoying the shakes and broth from time to time or as part of your daily regimen. They are both healthy and beneficial for the long term.

I would also recommend making the UltraBath part of your bedtime ritual to help you relax and sleep better.

However, the *single biggest gift you can give yourself at the end of this program is identifying which foods you are allergic to and which you can eat and enjoy safely.*

Reintroducing foods carefully as you transition out of the program can be a very useful and educational experience. If you do it properly, you will discover which foods have been making you sick and fat. You can then keep them out of your diet, and choose foods that make you thrive instead. Later you can expand your diet to include items you have eliminated.

The remainder of this chapter will focus on a step-by-step plan for reintroducing foods into your diet. I **strongly** encourage you to follow this plan. When you end the program, don't give up and go back to your old lifestyle. Maintain the vital health you have worked so hard to achieve and expand your understanding of how food works with your body by carefully reintroducing foods.

An Important Warning

As great as you will feel as the end of this program, you can feel ten times worse if you suddenly go back to your old habits.

Why does this happen?

Allergies result when a foreign protein (or antigen) joins with an antibody causing an immune or allergic reaction. When you eliminate the foods that produce allergies, the foreign proteins or antigens suddenly drop in your blood.

Then the antibodies have nothing to join on to, so you don't have an allergic reaction. This leads to the feeling of wellness and health you achieve at the end of the program.

You can get rid of these antigens quickly by not eating the problem foods. Unfortunately the antibodies to those foods take a few months to be eliminated by the body.

So when you suddenly eat that loaf of bread or hunk of cheese after your elimination diet, all those antibodies floating around in your blood gang up on the foreign proteins, leading to a sudden and dramatic allergic reaction we call serum sickness.

So *please* follow the food reintroduction guidelines below carefully, or you can feel worse than when you started. (Then again, that might be a good learning experience that will reinforce the power food has to make you feel great or horrible.)

Reintroduction of Potentially Allergenic Foods

After taking the "Toxicity and Inflammation Quiz" and the rest of your vitals, the next step is to start re-introducing the foods you eliminated during the program to see if any of them lead to symptoms or problems. This will allow you to identify problem foods, and avoid them for a longer period of time, to let your immune system cool off a little more.

Keep a log of any symptoms that you experience when you reintroduce different food groups. Remember, symptoms may occur anywhere from a few minutes to 72 hours after ingestion and can include fatigue, brain fog, mood changes, headaches, digestive upset, sleep problems, rashes, joint pains, fluid retention, and more.

Tracking your symptoms should guide you to which foods trigger allergic reactions in your system. When you identify the foods you are allergic to, it's best to avoid them for 90 days. Then you can reintroduce them again, but eat them no more than every 4 or 5 days.

Using a food log to track your symptoms and monitor your progress is an excellent way to identify what foods you can tolerate and what foods you are allergic to.

There is not enough room here to print a sample; however, I have included one in the downloadable *UltraSimple Companion Guide* at www.ultrasimplediet.com/guide. It is a very detailed food log that you can use to fill in the blanks quite easily.

Alternatively, I've also included this feature in our community at www.ultrasimplediet.com/join so you can track what you are eating online.

Note: Common symptoms may be postnasal drip, digestive problems such as bloating, gas, constipation or diarrhea, reflux, headaches, joint pains, fluid retention, fatigue, brain fog, mood changes, change in sleep pattern, rashes, and more.

Here is a plan for how to reintroduce foods over a few weeks so you can maximize the benefits of what you have just experienced.

Food Reintroduction

Phase One Reintroduction—2 Weeks

Foods or Ingredients to Permanently Avoid:

✧ High-fructose corn syrup
✧ Trans or hydrogenated fats
✧ Processed and junk foods
✧ Fast foods
✧ Artificial sweeteners
✧ Foods with additives, preservatives, and colors

Continue to Avoid in Phase One:

✧ Dairy (milk, cheese, butter, yogurt)
✧ Gluten (barley, rye, oats, spelt, kamut, triticale, wheat—see www.celiac.com for a complete list of foods that include gluten)
✧ Eggs
✧ Corn
✧ Peanuts

❖ Nightshades except chili peppers (tomatoes, egg-
   plants, bell peppers, potatoes)
❖ Citrus (except lemon)
❖ Caffeine
❖ Alcohol
❖ Sugars in any form (table sugar, honey, maple syrup,
   corn syrup)
❖ Yeasted products (wine, vinegar, breads)

Foods to add in Phase One:

❖ Fresh fruit (except citrus, pineapple, or dried fruit)
❖ Eat more raw vegetables like salads. Include artichokes, avocadoes, and olives.
❖ Organic lamb or beef, although you should keep
   these dense animal proteins to a minimum and consume no more than 4 ounces at a time. (You can find
   organic lamb, beef, and pork at Whole Foods Markets or online.)
❖ Grains: Add other low-allergy grains such as quinoa,
   buckwheat, millet.
❖ Continue to eat vegetables, beans, and rice.
❖ Healthy oils such as cold-pressed nut or seed oils in
   addition to the extra-virgin olive oil you have been
   using
❖ Spices: Continue to use garlic, ginger, curry or turmeric, rosemary, and fresh cilantro. In addition, you
   may now add any spices you enjoy.

When you eat out try:

❖ Japanese, Thai, Vietnamese, healthy Chinese (not
   fried, no MSG)

✦ Order fish and veggies at Italian restaurants.
✦ Avoid bread and desserts.

Phase Two Reintroduction

Add only one new food group every 3–4 days until you have added back all the foods you want to eat. This can take a while. Be patient. Doing this step by step will allow you to identify the problem foods for you within this list. If you experience symptoms from particular foods, you should avoid them for 90 days then try to introduce them again.

Add the foods back in the following order during Phase Two:

✦ Corn
✦ Peanuts
✦ Nightshades (tomatoes, eggplants, peppers, potatoes)
✦ Citrus
✦ Yeasted products (wine, vinegar, breads)
✦ Eggs
✦ Gluten (barley, rye, oats, spelt, kamut, wheat—see www.celiac.com for a complete list of foods that include gluten)
✦ Dairy (milk, cheese, butter, yogurt)
✦ Alcohol (only if you enjoy it in moderation)

When you reintroduce the top food allergens, eat them at least 2–3 times a day for 3 days to see if you notice a reaction (unless, of course, you notice a problem right away, then stop immediately).

As I recommended before, keep a log of common symptoms that can occur from a few minutes to 72 hours later. If you have a reaction, note the food and eliminate it for 90 days. This will give your immune system a chance to cool off and your gut a chance to heal. In turn, this makes it more likely you will be able to tolerate more foods in the long run. However, you may find it best to eat them only occasionally (not more than once every 3–4 days) to keep the immune system cooled off.

After you have eliminated the food for 90 days (or 12 weeks), try to it reintroduce again. If you still have symptoms, you may need to avoid this food long term.

What about Caffeine and Alcohol?

Other substances such as caffeine and alcohol can be used from time to time, but be aware that they are drugs and need to be used wisely and moderately.

Regular use of coffee can increase your stress hormones and deplete you over time. I find that most people have more energy after they stop coffee than when they were on it. It gives you a short boost, but you pay for it later.

Alcohol may also be enjoyed in moderation. (1–3 drinks a week. Hard liquor–1 ounce, wine–5 ounces, beer–10 ounces.) If you are allergic to yeast, sulfites, or gluten, it's best to avoid beer and wine. You can enjoy low-allergy drinks such as potato vodka or tequila.

You have given yourself an awesome gift by embarking on The UltraSimple Diet.

Congratulate yourself for learning things about your body that will lead you to your ideal weight and health for the long term.

Summary

◇ You can make many of the elements of this program part of your regular life. They will support your health over the long term.

◇ Be sure to reintroduce potentially allergic foods carefully. If not you can make yourself sicker, and you may fail to learn which are your real trigger foods—foods that should be eliminated for a full 12 weeks.

What's Next

Learn how to give yourself an UltraMetabolism permanently.

Give Yourself an UltraMetabolism Permanently!

At the end of the program, after eating healthful foods, supporting your body with supplements, nourishing yourself with yoga, meditation, and daily aerobic activity, and nurturing your spirit with loving friends and peaceful activities, you will have given your body the rest and renewal it has most likely been craving.

You will now be ready to start on a lifelong routine of healthy living based on the principles outlined and achieve UltraWellness. You will also have created the basis for preserving and supporting your health for a long time to come.

You have given yourself the wonderful gift of these 7 days. You have started on the road to vibrant health and have likely learned much about your body and your choices over the last 7 days. I congratulate you on taking this step in self-care.

Now that you have seen the power that 7 days of dietary and lifestyle change can have on your well-being and your waistline, I strongly encourage you to take the following three steps: make your UltraMetabolism permanent; share your success story; and help others reclaim their health.

Step 1: Make Your UltraMetabolism Permanent

Now that you've kick-started your metabolism, I encourage all of you to explore the full benefits of *UltraMetabolism: The*

Simple Plan for Automatic Weight Loss and learn how you may keep your revitalized health and weight loss permanent.

It is a book that's about losing weight, yes, but, more importantly, it's a user's manual for the human body that shows you how to optimize your health, which then naturally leads to weight loss. Based on decades of science and practice, it distills the fundamental knowledge of how your body works and breaks it down into step-by-step guidelines for you to achieve your full health potential and your optimal weight.

UltraMetabolism holds the keys to the healthy, thin person hiding inside of you. It can enable you to achieve lifelong health and permanent weight loss. No gimmicks. No tricks. Just simple, clear instructions based on a new medical paradigm that is revolutionizing medicine.

You don't have to wait decades to take advantage of the scientific advances that explain the basis of health and metabolism for the first time. We have all the information available now to solve this problem of obesity and chronic disease. You're just not hearing about it.

That's why I wrote *UltraMetabolism.*

One of the most common points of feedback I receive from people who have gone through this program was surprise at just how good modifying their diet made them feel.

They expected to starve themselves, eat bland food, count calories, and exercise all day only to have limited weight loss, but instead what they got was a simple plan that focused on eating delicious, nourishing foods that resulted not only in weight loss, but optimized health, better sleep, healthier, better-looking skin, more energy, better mood, and more.

This, of course, was not a surprise to me, as these results are what I've seen firsthand from many of my patients over the last two decades of doing this. But, just like with any eating plan, this is not a magic bullet that will result in permanent health and weight loss.

That is why I strongly recommend you take the next step, move on to the full UltraMetabolism program, which will give you the best shot at making your improvements over the last 7 days permanent and achieve UltraWellness.

You can get a free sneak preview of *UltraMetabolism* by going to www.ultrasimplediet.com/ultra

IMPORTANT: Some good news. Because you have already gone through this program, including the one-week preparation phase, you can jump immediately to week 2 of *UltraMetabolism* and skip week 1. It is not necessary to go through another preparation week since you've essentially already done that here.

Step #2: Share Your Success Story

One of my great joys in being a doctor is seeing the results of my recommendations firsthand, seeing people who previously had poor health all of sudden find themselves revitalized, and experiencing along with them their sheer happiness about their new lease on life.

While I can't see you personally, I would love to use the tools that the Web has given us so we can share in your success together virtually, online.

When you go to www.ultrasimplediet.com/success, you'll see hundreds of success stories from other people who have posted their results, pictures, and even videos. Not only are these incredibly satisfying for me to see, but they also provide the motivation and emotional encouragement that others need.

I would greatly appreciate it if you took just a few short moments to go to www.ultrasimplediet.com/success and share your success as well. You have the option of just leaving some comments or uploading before/after photos or videos if you like—it's completely up to you.

Even if you don't plan to share your own success story, I

encourage you to visit www.ultrasimplediet.com/success and to read those of others, both before starting the program and after, so you can see for yourself just how powerful this program is.

Step 3: Help Others Reclaim Their Health

One of the biggest challenges we face in defeating this obesity crisis is letting people know what programs work and what don't. My program isn't the only one out there, but if it does work for you, and it should, I would ask that you do the following:

Think of a loved one, a friend, coworker, associate, etc. who could use the help of this program. Let them know that they can get a free sneak preview of the program simply by going to www.ultrasimplediet.com/preview.

I will make certain parts of this book available for free, so they can get a taste of what this program is about. And hopefully you can share your own success story with them, so they can see firsthand how powerful this program can be.

It's simple: just have them go to www.ultrasimplediet.com/preview and they can instantly download a free sneak preview of this program.

That's it.

Congratulations on taking control of your health and caring for your body the way it was designed. You will feel the rewards now and for a long time to come—and most importantly, you are one step closer to achieving UltraWellness…a lifestyle of optimal health, full of energy, vitality, and happiness.

To your good health,

Mark Hyman, M.D.

ACKNOWLEDGMENTS

This book was not one I wanted to write. I don't believe in diets or dieting, but my patients and readers kept asking for something to get them started quickly. I thank them for helping me see the importance of laying out the principles of healing, detoxification, and dealing with inflammation and food allergies in a way that everyone can experience.

I learned these principles from my work with the Institute for Functional Medicine, Jeffrey Bland, and all the leaders, practitioners, and thinkers who have paved a new way for people with chronic disease to heal. I thank you all!

I also must thank all my staff at The UltraWellness Center who allow me to care for my patients AND do all the writing and teaching I also love to do. Especially Kathie Swift, who has taught me so much about food, healing, and how to help people change.

I especially must thank my UltraTeam, without whom I couldn't do half of what I can accomplish with them! Marc Stockman and Jeff Radich have found a way to help more and more people learn about new scientific discoveries in health, make everything accessible to so many, and take care of all the details big and small. Richard Pine, my agent, is a giant among men, thoughtful, encouraging, and passionately behind me. Sandi Mendelson, my publicist, is always there carrying the message out to the world for me!! And Spencer Smith helps me crystallize and organize my work into practical tools accessible to everyone—not an easy task. And my friends and supporters at Simon and Schuster, Scribner, and Pocket Books who believed in me from the beginning—Susan Moldow, Beth Wareham, Roz Lippel, Jack Romanos, Kevin Smith, Louise Burke, Abby Zidle, and Jean Ann Rose. I thank you all!

To help you get the most out of the UltraSimple program, you'll want to review these resources in addition to what's covered in this book:

- ✧ **The UltraSimple Community**—Here is where you can connect with others, share tips, advice, exchange recipes, record your private journal thoughts, track your health and weight and more. Go to www.ultra simplediet.com/join to join the community now.

- ✧ **The UltraSimple Companion Guide**—I've included lots of extra information that I didn't have room for in this book, including delicious recipes, helpful health and weight trackers, handy checklists, journal questions, a food log, FAQ, and a list of supplements that my patients typically take. Go to www .ultrasimplediet.com/guide to download this now.

- ✧ **UltraMetabolism Sneak Preview**—Once you are finished with the UltraSimple program, it's time to achieve lifelong UltraWellness by going through the advanced UltraMetabolism program. This is my *NY Times* best-selling book that reveals the full 8-week program that I typically put my patients through. Go to www.ultrasimplediet.com/ultra to download this free sneak preview now.

- ✧ **Seek Out UltraWellness**—Hopefully the success you've had on the UltraSimple program has given you a taste for how good you can really feel once you start working *with* your body instead of *against* it. The reality is that you have the ability to lead a vibrant, vivacious life full of vitality, happiness, and fulfillment, which can be yours once you achieve UltraWellness. To explore more about this, go to www.ultrawellness.com.

xxx

ABOUT THE AUTHOR

Mark Hyman, MD, is editor in chief of *Alternative Therapies in Health and Medicine,* the most prestigious journal in the field of Integrative Medicine, and the medical editor of *Alternative Medicine: The Art and Science of Healthy Living.* He is the coauthor of the *New York Times–*bestselling book published by Scribner, *Ultraprevention: The 6-Week Plan That Will Make You Healthy for Life,* and the author of *The Detox Box: A Program for Greater Health and Vitality,* recently published by Sounds True (2004) and the audio programs, *The Five Forces of Wellness: The Ultraprevention System for Living an Active, Age-Defying, Disease-Free Life* (Nightingale-Conant 2005), and *Nutrigenomics: The New Science of Health and Weight Loss* (2006). His latest book is the *New York Times* bestseller *UltraMetabolism: The Simple Plan for Automatic Weight Loss* (Scribner 2006). It focuses on a cutting-edge personalized—or "nutrigenomic"—approach to weight loss and metabolism. A companion PBS pledge special produced by WLIW features this approach.

A guest on the *Today* show, *Good Morning America, The Early Show,* and *The View* with Barbara Walters, Dr. Hyman has also appeared on CNN, FOX, PBS, and NPR, as well as many other television and radio stations. He has written for and is quoted regularly in leading consumer magazines including *Parade, Elle, Body and Soul, Fitness, Glamour, Family Circle, US, Women's World, First for Women, Health, Natural Health, Self, Shape,* and *Town & Country.*

For nearly 10 years, Dr. Hyman was the Co-Medical Director at Canyon Ranch Lenox, an internationally acclaimed

Health Resort. He is the founder and Medical Director of The
UltraWellness Center. His Web sites www.ultrawellness.com
and www.drhyman.com empower health care consumers and
allow them to take advantage of the medicine of the future, today. He is on the Board of Advisors and faculty of "Food as
Medicine" at the Center for Mind Body Medicine, Georgetown
University School of Medicine. He is also on the Board of Di-
rectors and faculty of the Institute for Functional Medicine and
collaborates with the Harvard Medical School's Division for
Research and Education in Complementary and Integrative
Medicine.

DOWNLOAD THE ULTRASIMPLE COMPANION
GUIDE TO BOOST YOUR SUCCESS

Although this book represents everything you'll need in order to successfully go through this program, I've put together a guide that you can download at no charge that includes several items that I didn't have enough room for in the book. To get the most out of the program, I suggest you download this guide before starting the program. The guide includes:

◇ **Delicious Recipes**—An expanded list of delicious recipes, including hot breakfast options, variations on the shake, tasty snack ideas and more that you can use during the program;

◇ **Helpful Trackers**—A handy set of charts so you can track how much your health and weight improves as you reduce your toxicity and inflammation during the program;

◇ **Handy Checklists**—A series of checklists that will allow you to easily keep track of all the steps you should taking during the preparation phase, the actual program itself, what to do afterward, shopping lists and more, so you can track the progress that you've made;

◇ **Journal Questions**—The list of daily journaling questions to help you relax and reflect with plenty of space for you to write your answers;

✧ **Food Log**—A detailed food log so you can track re-actions to foods you might be allergic to that might be making you toxic and inflamed;

✧ **FAQ**—Answers to the most commonly asked ques-tions that I've received on this program; if you have a question, chances are it's been answered in this portion;

✧ **Supplements**—A comprehensive list of supple-ments that I give to my patients in my private medi-cal practice, precise details for the type of ingredients you should look for and how to select high-quality brands, and a timing checklist for exactly when you should take these supplements.

To download the guide, simply go to:

http://www.ultrasimplediet.com/guide

In addition to the downloadable guide, I've put together a special website that includes many of the time-saving, program-enhancing tools that the guide has but that also allows you to connect with others on this program.

One of the wonderful things about the Internet is it allows me to stay in touch with many more people than I otherwise could. And at the same time it also allows all of you—people who are going through the same struggles and successes while losing weight and regaining your health—to stay in touch with each other.

When you join the UltraSimple community by going to www.ultrasimplediet.com/join, you'll get access to:

◈ **Recipe Exchange**—A recipe exchange so you can share your best recipes with others and search for delicious recipes that others have contributed;

◈ **Message Boards**—Message boards that allow you to connect with others to share advice and tips for getting the most out of the program;

◈ **Trackers**—An integrated module that allows you to track your health, weight, and other vital statistics all online, securely and privately;

◈ **Private Journal**—A private online journal where you can record your daily thoughts as well as a public blog that you can use to share thoughts with others;

✧ **Food Log**—A detailed food log so you can track reactions to foods you might be allergic to that might
be making you toxic and inflamed;

✧ **Share Your Success**—A place where you can post
your own success story and see and be motivated by
the hundreds of success stories posted by others;

✧ **Daily Encouragement**—Daily email reminders
during the 7-day program to keep you motivated and
on target

To join the UltraSimple community, please go to:

www.ultrasimplediet.com/join

Once you have finished the UltraSimple program, the next step on your path to achieving UltraWellness is to proceed to the UltraMetabolism program.

In this program, I unveil a groundbreaking but simple plan for automatic weight loss. Never before have all seven keys to permanent weight loss been integrated into a single plan.

Based on the cutting-edge science of nutrigenomics—the science of how food talks to our genes—UltraMetabolism promises to reprogram your body to automatically lose weight by turning on the messages of weight loss and health and turning off the messages of weight gain and disease.

Inside UltraMetabolism, you'll discover:

✦ Why you actually need to eat carbs to lose weight.— Page 41

✦ Why your body is designed to gain weight and what you can do to reprogram it to burn fat.—Page 3

✦ How several simple tests can pinpoint what's causing your weight-loss attempts to fail and what steps you can take to conquer the problems.—Page 80

✦ Why eating less and exercising more can actually make you fat.—Page 12

✦ How to control your appetite and feel full without counting carbs, fat, or calories.—Page 84

✧ How to turbo charge your metabolic furnace to burn extra fat while you sleep. (Do this one thing wrong and you'll actually force your body to pile on extra fat instead.)—Page 54

✧ Why this one special food could be your missing link to losing weight. (And why 95% of people don't get enough.)—Page 51

To download your free sneak preview, go to:

www.ultrasimplediet.com/ultra

Join Dr. Hyman's Weekly Blog

For more on the secrets to lifelong health and vitality join
Dr. Hyman's free weekly blog: **www.ultrawellness.com/blog**.

More books from Mark Hyman, M.D.

The UltraMind Solution: Fix Your Broken Brain by Healing Your Body First

Enhance mood, sharpen focus, overcome
anxiety and debilitating conditions.

Download a sneak preview:
www.ultrawellness.com/ums_sneak

UltraMetabolism: The Simple Plan for Automatic Weight Loss

Awaken the hidden fat-burning code in your
DNA and reprogram your metabolism

Download a sneak preview:
www.ultrawellness.com/um_sneak

The UltraMetabolism Cookbook: 200 Delicious Recipes for Automatic Weight Loss

Target your belly fat and boost energy.

Download a sneak preview:
www.ultrawellness.com/cookbook_sneak

UltraPrevention: The 6-Week Plan That Will Make You Healthy for Life (Co-authored by Dr. Hyman)

Discover the 5 principles for
restoring and maintaining health.

More at:
www.ultrawellness.com/up

Available wherever books are sold or at www.simonandschuster.com

Audio/Video Programs

Six Weeks to an UltraMind

A personalized 6-week, audio/video coaching program designed to heal your brain by fixing imbalances in your body's underlying biology.

More at: www.ultrawellness.com/six

UltraMind Subscription Club

A self-paced 9-week brain-boosting community designed to defeat depression, anxiety, and sharpen your mind.

More at: www.ultrawellness.com/sub

UltraMind Solution DVD

Watch as Dr. Hyman explains how to fix your mind by healing your body first.

More at: www.ultrawellness.com/ums_dvd

The Ultra Thyroid Solution

Pinpoint the hidden causes of your hypothyroidism.

More at: www.ultrawellness.com/ultra_thyroid

The 5 Forces of Wellness

Discover how your body works to stay well and live healthy.

More at: www.ultrawellness.com/forces

The Detox Box

Everything you need to complete a safe, effective, and medically informed detoxification program.

More at: www.ultrawellness.com/detoxbox